Hyperbaric Medicine

Vishal Mago

Hyperbaric Medicine

Recent Advances and Clinical Scenarios

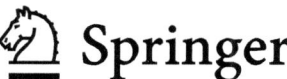 Springer

Vishal Mago
Professor and HOD, Department of Burn
and Plastic Surgery
AIIMS
Rishikesh, Uttarakhand, India

ISBN 978-981-95-2643-7   ISBN 978-981-95-2644-4   (eBook)
https://doi.org/10.1007/978-981-95-2644-4

This Springer imprint is published by the registered company Springer Nature Singapore Pte Ltd.
The registered company address is: 152 Beach Road, #21-01/04 Gateway East, Singapore 189721,
Singapore

If disposing of this product, please recycle the paper.

Foreword

In the evolving landscape of modern medicine, few disciplines remain as uniquely positioned at the crossroads of physiology, physics, and patient recovery as Hyperbaric Oxygen Therapy (HBOT). What began as a niche adjunct has, over decades, established itself as a lifesaving intervention and a vital component of the multidisciplinary continuum of care—especially in the management of complex wounds, radiation injuries, osteomyelitis, and hypoxic tissue syndromes.

This book is not only a reflection of that clinical transformation but also a call to action—a call to elevate hyperbaric medicine through rigorous inquiry, open collaboration, and a shared commitment to growing the clinical evidence base. My journey through this field has confirmed a central truth: hyperbaric medicine is only as powerful as the science that supports it and the clinicians who understand its potential.

As a practicing physician and educator, I have had the privilege of witnessing first-hand how HBOT can rescue ischemic tissue, reverse radiation necrosis, salvage limbs, and restore dignity to patients for whom conventional therapies have failed. Yet, the challenge that remains is not only delivering this care—it is explaining it, studying it, publishing it, and sharing it across specialties, borders, and generations of clinicians.

The importance of a unified, evidence-driven hyperbaric community has never been greater. As technology evolves, so too must our standards, protocols, and outcomes data. This book is my contribution to that effort—a platform for clinical insights, case-based learning, and practical applications of HBOT that I hope will serve as a catalyst for thoughtful discussion and deeper investigation. I applaud Dr. Mago for his dedication in the field of Hyperbarics.

Each chapter has been crafted not only to educate but to invite dialogue—to bridge the gap between theory and bedside, between skeptics and advocates, between early-career practitioners and seasoned hyperbaric professionals. My intent is to shine a light on the remarkable versatility of HBOT and to explore its use as more than a modality—but as a philosophy of care grounded in tissue physiology, interprofessional collaboration, and patient-centered outcomes.

I firmly believe that the future of hyperbaric medicine lies in our willingness to question, to document, to publish, and to push forward together. That future is not dictated by reimbursement tables or regulatory challenges but by the strength of our clinical data, the courage of our ideas, and the patients whose lives are changed every day by this therapy.

To those who seek to understand more, to practice better, and to lead boldly—I welcome you to this work. May it serve as both a guide and a spark. Congratulations!

American College of Hyperbaric Medicine   Tyler Sexton
Austin, TX, USA

Contents

Chapter 1
History of Hyperbaric Medicine

History of Chamber

The use of hyperbaric oxygen in patient therapy dates back to the seventeenth century, when C. Henshaw, a British physician and physiologist, designed the first hyperbaric chamber known as Domicilium. I. Boerema, a Dutch surgeon, is considered to be the father of modern oxygen hyperbaric oxygen therapy. He advocated not to use pressures more than 3 atmospheres absolute [1]. John Scott Haldane is considered as the father of decompression sickness. His methods form the basis for treating bends. Haldane gave the concept of half saturation of nitrogen gas.

In 1775, Joseph Priestley discovered the role of oxygen and Lavoisier coined the term "oxygen." Paul Bert, considered as "the father of hyperbaric physiology" (1878), gave the concept of oxygen toxicity and his work was labeled as the Bert Effect, i.e., central nervous system toxicity due to exposure of oxygen more than 1.6 bars. The effects of water pressure on the body was demonstrated [2].

The French surgeon Fontaine built a mobile pressurized operating room in 1879. In 1928, Oliver Cunningham made the Silver Ball hospital which had 6 stories and reached a pressure of 3 atmospheres. This was closed in 1930 due to lack of evidence. US treatment tables were made in 1954. Behnke and Shaw(1937) first used hyperbaric medicine to treat decompression sickness in deep-sea divers.

The patients of carbon monoxide poisoning were treated by hyperbaric in 1962. The patients of gas gangrene were treated by hyperbaric medicine with a mortality of 11.1% [3]. Undersea Hyperbaric society was started in the USA in Maryland in 1967 to conduct instructional courses on hyperbaric oxygen therapy. In 1980, a Divers alert network(DAN) was established with help of UHMS to provide emergency services for divers.

In 1989, European Committee of hyperbaric medicine took shape.

The dive limit for oxygen toxicity was evident in the era of World War II, where submarine technology was evolving along with modifications in mine workers

V. Mago, *Hyperbaric Medicine*, https://doi.org/10.1007/978-981-95-2644-4_1

breathing apparatuses. This apparatus was modified for using it underwater subsequently. This paved the way for the establishment of diving safety guidelines and hyperbaric facility safety for diving accidents. German and Dutch societies played an important role in the development of dive medicine.

Hyperbaric and Surgery

Dr. Christian Barnard used hyperbaric therapy in congenital heart disease. Dr. Davidson used hyperbaric in irradiation cancer patients. Dr. Boerema is considered the messiah of hyperbaric surgery. He performed animal experiments in Don helder hyperbaric tank. In 1959, they built a steel chamber, where they demonstrated that oxygen content increases 20 times if inhaled at a pressure of 3 atmospheres. In 1974, a hyperbaric center with 6 multiplace chambers was built in Moscow where 1000 cardiac and vascular surgeries were performed. Keogh reported the first case of clostridial brain abscess treated with hyperbaric oxygen [4]. Still further articles elucidated and potentiated the role of this therapy in management of gas gangrene.

Three hyperbaric-oxygen treatments within a 24-hour period plays a major role in reducing cognitive sequel 6 weeks and 12 months after acute carbon monoxide poisoning [5].

The three main gases in relation to Hyperbaric oxygen therapy are oxygen, nitrogen, and carbon dioxide. Various gas laws related to how pressure of a gas changes with concentration within tissues has been well documented.

Studies on the role of hyperbaric oxygen in wounds is widely covered in the literature. Increased oxygenation promotes fibroblast proliferation [6].

To date, a lot of new discoveries have been made in hyperbaric with the addition of 14 indications by UHMS and pressures of less than 2 ATA are found useful in neurological indications.

Equipment Functionality

The European code of good clinical practice for HBOT ensures the minimum requirements for quality issues of working of the equipment based on European standards. The risk evaluations are performed periodically for the chambers. UHMS has released guidelines for working of hyperbaric chambers. Nayional Fire Protection Association 99 has given fire safety guidelines in these chambers. The American Society of Mechanical Engineers(ASME) has established certification of these chambers and Compressed Gas Association provides parameters for handling of medical gases.

Chambers in India/Abroad

The Indian subcontinent has seen installation of around 50 hyperbaric centers till date. The companies manufacturing hyperbaric chambers are Sechrist, Tekna, and Perry. In 1981, Perry Baromedical installed the first multiplace chamber in British Columbia hospital, Canada and delivered the first acrylic multiplace chamber to St Mary's hospital, Florida(1986). Tekna Limited is in business since 1989 with the manufacture of both class A-multiplace, B-monoplace, and C animal chambers in India. It is providing sales, service, and training in hyperbaric therapy. Sechrist industries are manufacturing H series hyperbaric chambers under guidance of Ron Sechrist since 1973. Baromedic health care in Pune has installed chambers all over India. Cuba has almost 50 hyperbaric chambers whereas Mexico houses a total of 124 chambers. Neurological indications are treated in hyperbaric chambers of Japan. It is also highly developed in China, Turkey, Korea, and Australia. In Spain, the Centre for Underwater Recovery and Research(CRIS) treating patients of decompression sickness is the oldest center since 1954. This paved the way for safe treatment of diving accidents [7]. UHMS gave the approval of use of HBOT in burns in 1989. Hart and others demonstrated decreased requirements of intravenous fluids and rapid wound healing rates with HBOT [8].

References

1. Boerema I. The use of hyperbaric oxygen. Am Heart J. 1965;69:289–92.
2. Raymond KA, Cooper JS. Scuba diving physiology. In: StatPearls [Internet]. Treasure Island (FL): StatPearls Publishing; 2025.
3. Fowler DL, Evans LL, Mallow JE. Monoplace hyperbaric oxygen therapy for gas gangrene. JAMA. 1977;238(8):882–3.
4. Keogh AJ. Clostridial brain abscess and hyperbaric oxygen. Postgrad Med J. 1973;49(567):64–6. https://doi.org/10.1136/pgmj.49.567.64.
5. Weaver LK, Hopkins RO, Chan KJ, Churchill S, Elliott CG, Clemmer TP, Orme JF Jr, Thomas FO, Morris AH. Hyperbaric oxygen for acute carbon monoxide poisoning. N Engl J Med. 2002;347(14):1057–67.
6. Tompach PC, Lew D, Stoll JL. Cell response to hyperbaric oxygen treatment. Int J Oral Maxillofac Surg. 1997;26(2):82–6.
7. Maroni A. The XIII annual Chinese symposium on hyperbaric medicine. Foundation Int Congress Hyperbar Med. 2004;6(2):6–6.
8. Weiss LD, Van Meter KW. The applications of hyperbaric oxygen therapy in emergency medicine. Am J Emerg Med. 1992;10(6):558–68.

Chapter 2
Types of Chambers

Introduction

Hyperbaric oxygen therapy is provided by:

1. Breathing oxygen through mask or bib.
2. Increased barometric pressure.
3. Mono or multiplace chamber.

There are 2 types of hyperbaric chambers:

A. Monoplace.

Single vessel compartment for single patient (Fig. 2.1).

B. Multiplace.

They have 2 or more compartments for more than 2 patients at a time (Fig. 2.2). These chambers are further classified as low (<2.5 bar), medium (2.5–5 bars), or high (>5 Bar). Based on working capability, it can be classified as oxygen only or breathing mixture of gases. These systems should be US FDA or CE approved. The operational safety of these chambers are governed by NFPA and ASME. The American Society of Mechanical Engineers and Pressure Vessels of Human Occupancy established guidelines for the design and construction of these chambers.

V. Mago, *Hyperbaric Medicine*, https://doi.org/10.1007/978-981-95-2644-4_2

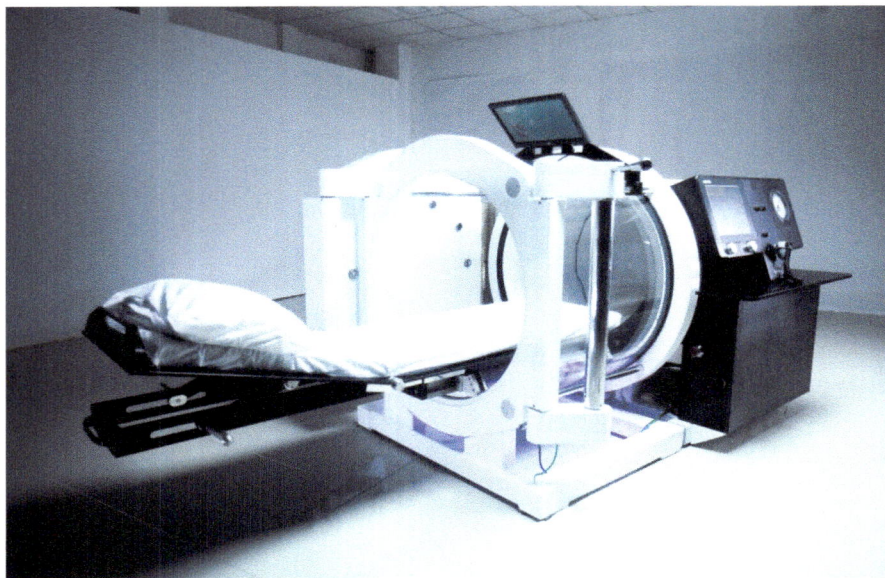

Fig. 2.1   Tekna monoplace chamber

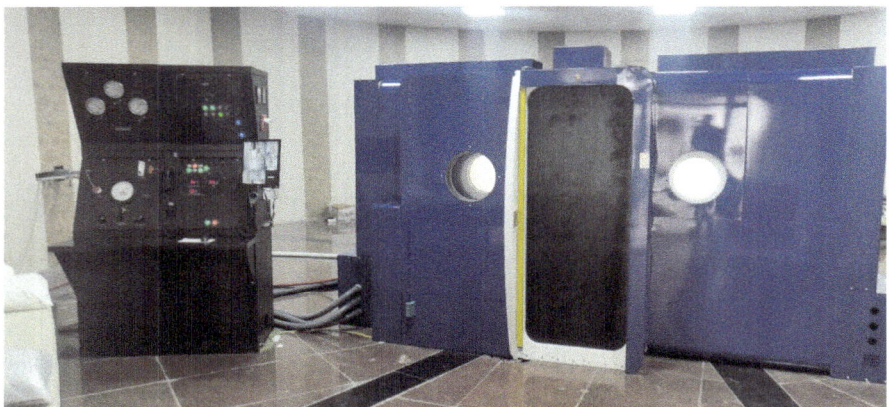

Fig. 2.2   Multiplace hyperbaric chamber

Monoplace Chambers

These are single compartment vessels providing hyperbaric oxygen to single patient with maximum operational pressure of 200 kPa (2 bar). These chambers have a clear tube made of acrylic glass allowing the patient to see outside with safety features like communication systems,door lock and gas monitoring system, Treatment times are 60–90 minutes, depending on the indications. It can be transportable or fixed. Oxygen flows to the device are through face mask during active treatment to avoid CO_2 accumulation. To initiate an air break, the chamber operator switches the face tent's oxygen supply to air and reverts to oxygen upon completion of the air break. These chambers are also found at dive sites near diving operations. The disadvantages of this chamber are patient isolation, claustrophobia, and lack of invasive monitoring. Drugs can be passed easily through epidural catheters [2]. Better hygiene practices can be inculcated and useful in awake children. The financial issues incurred on treatment are less. The minimum staff to run a monoplace is one hyperbaric physician or surgeon, attendant, and nursing technician.

Multiplace Hyperbaric Chamber

These are chambers with one or more compartments with an air lock device for door closure. The oxygen is given by masks or bibs or endotracheal tubes. The advantages of a multiplace chamber are more patients can be accommodated, low risk of claustrophobia, less risk of infection, and better management of critical patient. It provides an eye-to-eye contact with the technician inside the chamber and nursing supervision is available. There are more chances of manipulating US Navy tables with variable pressures. Immediate medical treatment can be provided in an emergency and machine can be halted by pressing emergency lever. The Maquet Servo i Ventilator is compatible with hyperbaric chamber [3]. The multiplace chamber is better equipped to manage critical ICU patients and Hospira Plum A infusion pump can be used inside a pressurized chamber [4].

The implantable devices can malfunction in a hyperbaric chamber and so should be avoided [5]. Use of defibrillation devices are to be avoided in a multiplace chamber [6].

The parts of a hyperbaric chamber are:

A. Pressure vessel with acrylic windows.
B. Patient access hatches with viewports.
C. An airlock for door.
D. Small access for passing medicines or instruments.
E. Air pressurisation system with CCTV monitors.

Chamber Room

Placing the containers on the ground floor in a secluded area free from fire risks is important. The room housing the chamber should be big enough to lodge the multiplace unit with its compressor and backup unit. Chamber flooring should be made of non combustible material and be positively grounded. Penetrators should be designed for gas/fluid interchange separated from electric connections. Excessive chamber partitions or proximity of ventilation terminals are to be kept in mind while designing these chambers.

Fire Protection

The chambers have built-in antistatic points to prevent pile up of electrical charge. Adequate number of grade A fire extinguishers must be in place all around the chamber. There are "No Smoking" signboards displayed all around in the vicinity of the facility. The patients are instructed to wear cotton clothes before entering the chamber. The patients cannot use spirit-based handwashing solutions. In the event of a fire, adequate escape plans should be in place and light backup systems should be in standby modes. Defibrillation should be avoided in a chamber to mitigate fire risk [6]. Compressing the chamber with air reduces risk of explosion.

Gas Supply

Medical grade oxygen is delivered inside the chamber through use of face masks, bibs, or endotracheal tubes to maintain safe oxygen levels. The quality of air inside the chamber has carbon dioxide levels <5000 ppm and oxygen concentration of <23.5%. Most hyperbaric chambers use air as the pressurization air for achieving a specified hyperbaric ventilation rate of 30 actual liters per minute(alpm) per person [1].

How to Choose an Adequate Chamber

The pressure containers should be chosen based on ASME PVHO 1 standards. The number of bunkers or lifts or gurney is decided by its proper design and construction, ensuring proper design of piping and storage shelves. Most clinical hyperbaric chambers can withstand pressures of up to 6 atmospheres.

Windows should be in accordance with ASME PVHO standards based on the design of chambers. Internal mounted CCTV cameras should be in place in modern chambers. A rectangular door is ideal to provide easy access of patients and gurneys. There should be a minimum number of penetrators per compartment.

The chamber paint and primers are fire resistant, durable, and non-toxic to people sitting inside the chamber. Undesirable odors are prohibited inside these chambers.

Seats and Bunks

They are made up of non-combustible and non-sparking material and must be grounded.

Beds and Trolleys.

The bearings used on trolleys are lubricant free.

The SOPS (standard operating procedures) have been defined and are in place for working and management of hyperbaric chambers in our hospitals for ensuring the safety and quality of the devices. These include:

1. Conducting daily chamber sessions as per the indications.
2. Use of door locks.
3. Recording of sessions on proforma.
4. Shut down work mechanism.
5. Management of gas supply.
6. Cleaning and disinfection of chamber.
7. Use of all other medical devices.
8. Treatment protocols.
9. Patient preparation and PAC checkup.
10. Team role.
11. Record keeping.
12. Incident report of adverse events.
13. System failure record.
14. Annual maintenance record of the system.

References

1. Matity L, Burman F, Kot J, Caruana J. Effectiveness of hyperbaric chamber ventilation. Diving Hyperb Med. 2023;53(2):85–91.
2. Lind F. A pro/con review comparing the use of mono- and multiplace hyperbaric chambers for critical care. Diving Hyperb Med. 2015;45(1):56–60.
3. Weaver LK. Operational use and patient care in the monoplace hyperbaric chamber. Respir Care Clin N Am. 1999;5(1):51–92.
4. Millar IL. Hyperbaric intensive care technology and equipment. Diving Hyperb Med. 2015;45:50–6.
5. Bell J, Weaver LK, Deru K. Performance of the Hospira plum a+ (HB) hyperbaric infusion pump. Undersea Hyperb Med. 2014;41(3):235–43.
6. Kot J. Medical devices and procedures in the hyperbaric chamber. Diving Hyperb Med. 2014;44(4):223–7.

Chapter 3
Physics of Hyperbaric Medicine and Oxygen Metabolism

Introduction

Oxygen is used as a drug in hyperbaric therapy to perform the various functions of metabolism leading to its beneficial role in various indications. It plays a radio-sensitizing role at pressures of 1.9 to 2.5 ATA.

The human body is compartmentalized to perform gas exchange at various levels to supply oxygen from inspired gas in the lungs to the cells where mitochondria play a crucial role in cell respiration. The red blood cells in micro-circulation pick up the oxygen from the atmosphere and deliver it to the rest of the body by the action of the left side of the heart. The blood plasma has a large oxygen carrying capacity which carries oxygen to peripheral cells especially in the brain, heart, and eyes.

Hyperbaric therapy increases oxygen (35–40%) in the body especially oxygen dissolved in blood plasma. Table 3.1 depicts the beneficial effects of hyperbaric oxygen therapy on metabolic diseases and clinical scenarios.

Simultaneous sessions of hyperbaric oxygen treatments in the postischemic phase stimulate aerobic metabolism in muscle. Mild hyperbaric oxygen inhibits decrease in dopaminergic neurons in Parkinson's disease [1].

The mechanism through which hyperbaric therapy improves microcirculation in diabetes and radiation injuries is effective increase in the radius of oxygen diffusion in capillaries. It improves interstitial edema which is detrimental in cases of radiation fibrosis.

The uptake and transport of oxygen in ischemic zones increases due to an increase in oxygen concentration. Hyperoxic vasoconstriction accentuates the vaso-motion and vascular bypass beneficial in ischemic tissues. Hyperbaric oxygen leads to an increase in HIF stimulating angiogenesis preventing damage to intestine, lungs, brain, and heart.

V. Mago, *Hyperbaric Medicine*, https://doi.org/10.1007/978-981-95-2644-4_3

Table 3.1 Metabolic effects of hyperbaric oxygen

Metabolic disease	Target person/ organ	Effects	References
Type 2 diabetes	Humans	Decreased fasting blood glucose by 19% and increased whole-body, hepatic, and increased insulin sensitivity by about one third	[2]
DNA damage	Human lymphocytes	Low-level overexpression of heme oxygenase provides protection against oxidative DNA damage induced by HBO	[3]
Hypoglycemia	Human diabetic patients	The incidence of hypoglycemia (defined as $\leq$70 mg/dL) during or immediately after HBO2 treatment was 1.5%	[4]
Hypertension	Rats	The hyperbaric group of WKY rats exhibited lower SBP than the age-matched normobaric group	[5]
Male infertility	Human male patients	15 embryos were obtained in the globozoospermic group, which was the highest number, 10 were obtained from the azoospermic patients in assisted reproductive treatment	[6]
Traumatic brain injury	Human patients	HBOT can induce neuroplasticity leading to repair of chronically impaired brain functions and improved quality of life in mTBI patients	[7]
Muscle	Rats	Repeated hyperbaric oxygen treatments in the postischemic phase stimulate aerobic metabolism	[8]
Aging	Humans	Following HBOT, there was a significant increase in collagen density ($p < 0.001$, effect size(es) = 1.10), elastic fiber length ($p < 0.0001$, es = 2.71), and the number of blood vessels ($p = 0.02$, es = 1.00) in biopsy specimens	[9]

Effects of HBO in Diabetes Mellitus

Hyperbaric therapy induces metabolic changes and microcirculatory changes after ten sessions in diabetic foot ulcers with a decrease in the size of ulcers and promotion of granulation on wound bed. Low dose reactive oxygen species mitohormesis and increase in mitochondrial capacity leads to improvement of insulin sensitivity[2].Hypoglycemia is seen in HBO sessions with Type 1 diabetes [4].

Hyperbaric therapy reduces levels of very-low-density lipoprotein (VLDL), intermediate-density lipoprotein (IDL 3), LDL 1, LDL 2, and LDL 3. Glycemic activity also improves with this therapy [10].

The mechanism by which hyperbaric oxygen therapy improves micro-circulation in diabetic patients is by antiatherogenic, antioxidant, and cardioprotective effects. HBOT regulates molecules of nitric oxide synthesis that exerts anti-inflammatory and angiogenic effects in patients with DM [11].

Hyperbaric oxygen therapy increased the healing rate of diabetic foot ulcers in 17 studies, shortened the healing time, and reduced the incidence of major amputation. The anxiety levels were lowered following therapy [12].

Principles

The principles are based on certain gas laws:

1. Henry.
2. Fick.
3. Boyle.
4. Dalton.

Henry's Law

It states that the concentration of dissolved gas is equal to pressure times the solubility coefficient of that gas.

This law is applicable in opening a can of Pepsi, the carbon dioxide escapes into the atmosphere. Once the partial pressure of carbon dioxide decreases in the atmosphere, the carbon dioxide level in the Pepsi can also decrease.

This law plays an important role in respiration of gases as concentration of dissolved carbon dioxide is very high in deoxygenated blood so the gas moves from blood to alveoli in the lungs. This law proves useful in management of CO poisoning,crush injuries and anemia.

Fick's Law

It states that movement of solute occurs from a higher to a lower concentration. This explains the physiologic basis in gas bubble reduction in decompression sickness or its beneficial role in antimicrobial activity. Diabetic foot ulcer explains usefulness of this law by increase in pressure gradient to 2000mmHg in hypoxic tissues drives oxygen to promote angiogenesis,collagen synthesis and bactericidal effects.

Boyle's Law

This law states that the volume of a gas is inversely proportional to its pressure. This is attributed to the role of hyperbaric in Caisson's disease, leading to a reduction in size of bubbles at pressures of 3 ATA. The size of bubbles reduce to two thirds in size with therapy. The complications of ear or pulmonary barotrauma exemplifies this law. This testifies why the volume of gases increase during decompression phase of the chamber. A diver with nitrogen bubbles can improve with HBOT by compression and removal of bubbles.

Dalton's Law

It states that the total pressure of a mixture of gases is equal to partial pressure of individual gases. High oxygen pressures are delivered to the lung inside a chamber with increase in chamber pressure. It eliminates nitrogen from inspired air and drives more oxygen into the tissues.It helps in oxygen toxicity management.

Physiology

The air we breathe contains 21% oxygen. The oxygen is carried by blood in two ways

1. Hemoglobin.
2. Plasma.

Hemoglobin carries the majority of the oxygen as compared to plasma. One hundred ml of blood carries 19 ml of oxygen as hemoglobin and 0.32 ml oxygen in plasma. As the pressure increases in a chamber, i.e., at 2ATA this value becomes 4.4 ml/dl. This hyper-oxygenation leads to a plethora of effects in the form of angiogenesis, leukocyte oxidative killing, fibroblast proliferation, and toxin inhibition. An exercising muscle is hot, acidic, and hypercarbic, as this benefit is due to oxygen extraction from capillaries.

Hyperoxia in normal tissues causes vasoconstriction which results in reduction of edema in burns and compartment syndrome. Oxygen is vital for cross-linking and maturation of collagen along with hydroxylation of lysine.

Hyperbaric increases the oxygen gradient, thereby promoting angiogenesis. Fibroblast proliferation leads to revascularization in tissues. HBOT restores aerobic respiration.It stimulates anti oxidant enzyme production.

Direct bactericidal effects occur inside a chamber by generation of free radicals. HIF-1 and HIF-2 regulate the transcriptional response to hypoxia. Under hypoxic conditions, there is a reduction in oxygen and ROS molecules, HIF-1α sub units are not hydrolyzed, which generate the active HIF transcription factor. At the hyperoxic environment, more ROS and oxygen are available; thus more HIF-1α subunits are hydrolyzed [13]. There is a peak in levels of reactive oxygen species at 1.4 ATA and 2.5 ATA in healthy volunteers seen at 48 hours after the sessions [14]. There was an increase in plasma catalase and neopterin which activates the immune system. Neopterin is a neuroprotective agent which improves cognitive performance in traumatic brain injury patients. Figure 3.1 exemplifies the role of hypoxia in different clinical scenarios.

Fig. 3.1 Role of hypoxia
in different conditions

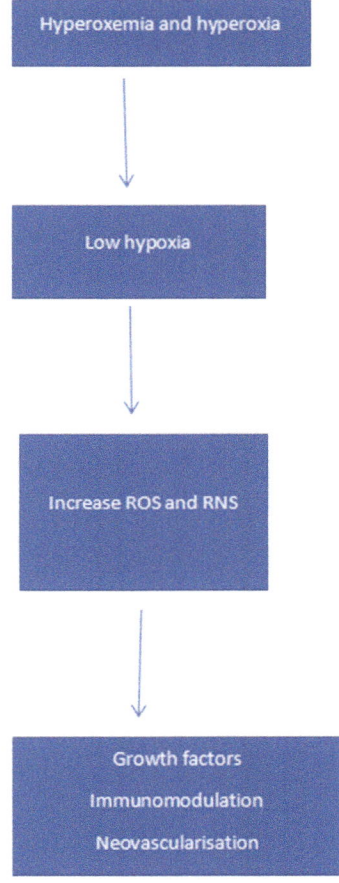

A change in oxygen level at cellular level leads to a cascade of events due to hypoxia while intermittent hyperoxia generates a tissue regenerative response known as the "hyperoxic hypoxic paradox." Intermittent hyperoxia is achieved by hyperbaric therapy. The arterial oxygen tension reaches 1500 mm Hg and tissue levels of 200–400 mmHg. VEGF production is stimulated by HIF 1 leading to angiogenesis and improves blood flow in ischemic tissues in patients of peripheral arterial disease. In hyperbaric, elevated pressure and elevated oxygen increases matrix mineralization at levels higher than those seen in normobaric controls. Ironically the increment in extracellular calcium deposition was already evident after 14 days of culture [15]. Gas solubility and diffusion gradients based on Henry's and Dalton's laws play an important role in nitrogen narcosis and bends associated with decompression sickness syndrome.

Oxygen is a significant factor in wound healing. Acute wounds are hypoxic and simulates extraction of oxygenated plasma in hypoxic tissue and promotes healing. Oxygen is an energy source for cell function. It acts as a cofactor for NO and hydrogen peroxide. It is a substrate for ROS which helps in eradicating infection. It plays a role in redox switch and promotes angiogenesis by increasing levels of VEGF from fibroblasts and macrophages. Most of the clinical protocols in HBOT are programmed to maximize beneficial effects of ROS/RNS in clinical scenarios while avoiding oxygen toxicity.

References

1. Ishihara A. Mild hyperbaric oxygen: mechanisms and effects. J Physiol Sci. 2019;69(4):573–80.
2. Sarabhai T, Mastrototaro L, Kahl S, Bönhof GJ, Jonuscheit M, Bobrov P, Katsuyama H, Guthoff R, Wolkersdorfer M, Herder C, Meuth SG, Dreyer S, Roden M. Hyperbaric oxygen rapidly improves tissue-specific insulin sensitivity and mitochondrial capacity in humans with type 2 diabetes: a randomised placebo-controlled crossover trial. Diabetologia. 2023;66(1):57–69.
3. Rothfuss A, Speit G. Overexpression of heme oxygenase-1 (HO-1) in V79 cells results in increased resistance to hyperbaric oxygen (HBO)-induced DNA damage. Environ Mol Mutagen. 2002;40(4):258–65.
4. Stevens SL, Narr AJ, Claus PL, Millman MP, Steinkraus LW, Shields RC, Buchta WG, Haddon R, Wang Z, Murad MH. The incidence of hypoglycemia during HBO2 therapy: a retrospective review. Undersea Hyperb Med. 2015;42(3):191–6.
5. Nagatomo F, Fujino H, Takeda I, Ishihara A. Effects of hyperbaric oxygenation on blood pressure levels of spontaneously hypertensive rats. Clin Exp Hypertens. 2010;32(3):193–7.
6. Özgök Kangal K, Özgök Y. Assisted reproductive treatments with hyperbaric oxygen therapy in male infertility. Turk J Urol. 2021;47(2):98–105.
7. Boussi-Gross R, Golan H, Fishlev G, Bechor Y, Volkov O, Bergan J, Friedman M, Hoofien D, Shlamkovitch N, Ben-Jacob E, Efrati S. Hyperbaric oxygen therapy can improve post concussion syndrome years after mild traumatic brain injury – randomized prospective trial. PLoS One. 2013;8(11):e79995.
8. Nylander G, Nordström H, Lewis D, Larsson J. Metabolic effects of hyperbaric oxygen in postischemic muscle. Plast Reconstr Surg. 1987;79(1):91–7.
9. Hachmo Y, Hadanny A, Mendelovic S, Hillman P, Shapira E, Landau G, Gattegno H, Zrachya A, Daniel-Kotovsky M, Catalogna M, Fishlev G, Lang E, Polak N, Doenyas K, Friedman M, Zemel Y, Bechor Y, Efrati S. The effect of hyperbaric oxygen therapy on the pathophysiology of skin aging: a prospective clinical trial. Aging (Albany NY). 2021;13(22):24500–10.
10. Balaz D, Komornikova A, Sabaka P, Leichenbergova E, Leichenbergova K, Novy M, Kralikova D, Gaspar L, Dukat A. Changes in vasomotion – effect of hyperbaric oxygen in patients with diabetes type 2. Undersea Hyperb Med. 2016;43(2):123–34.
11. Resanović I, Zarić B, Radovanović J, Sudar-Milovanović E, Gluvić Z, Jevremović D, Isenović ER. Hyperbaric oxygen therapy and vascular complications in diabetes mellitus. Angiology. 2020;71(10):876–85.
12. Zhang Z, Zhang W, Xu Y, Liu D. Efficacy of hyperbaric oxygen therapy for diabetic foot ulcers: an updated systematic review and meta-analysis. Asian J Surg. 2022;45(1):68–78.
13. Hadanny A, Efrati S. The hyperoxic-hypoxic paradox. Biomolecules. 2020;10(6):958.
14. Leveque C, Mrakic Sposta S, Theunissen S, Germonpré P, Lambrechts K, Vezzoli A, Bosco G, Lévénez M, Lafère P, Guerrero F, Balestra C. Oxidative stress response kinetics after 60 minutes at different (1.4 ATA and 2.5 ATA) hyperbaric hyperoxia exposures. Int J Mol Sci. 2023;24(15):12361.
15. Lin SS, Ueng SW, Niu CC, Yuan LJ, Yang CY, Chen WJ, Lee MS, Chen JK. Effects of hyperbaric oxygen on the osteogenic differentiation of mesenchymal stem cells. BMC Musculoskelet Disord. 2014;15:56. https://doi.org/10.1186/1471-2474-15-56.

Chapter 4
Ischemia Reperfusion Injury in Hyperbaric Medicine

Introduction

The methods used to reduce ischemia reperfusion injury are antioxidants to reduce oxidative stress, free radical scavengers to remove metabolic waste, and hypoxic preconditioning. Within 6 hours of onset of insult if HBOT is used, it reverses the local hypoxia, reduces edema, preserves penumbra of injury, and enhances survival of organs. Ischemia-Reperfusion Injury (IRI) is a complication following the reperfusion of ischemic tissues.

Types of injuries based on Ischemia reperfusion:

1. Traumatic brain injury.
2. Thermal burns.
3. Embolic or thrombolytic disorders.
4. Organ transplant.
5. Replantation.

The severity of IRI depends upon the following factors:

1. Duration of ischemia.
2. Size of infarct.
3. Function of tissue.

Brain shows irreversible injury if treatment is delayed by 20 min. Hyperbaric limits infarct size in reperfused animal heart studies. Intestines are highly vulnerable followed by skeletal muscle which if >4 hours rhabdomyolysis ensues.

Pathophysiology

IRI patterns of injury are a conglomerate of similar pathologic processes. These common factors are:

1. Oxidative stress.
2. ROS activity.
3. Inflammation.
4. Increased neutrophil endothelial cell interaction.
5. Microvascular dysfunction.

Patients with traumatic amputations or stroke experience life-threatening complications even after the main injuries have been aborted. It is essential to monitor the patient's condition post-replantation, as the restoration of blood flow to ischemic tissues can lead to reperfusion injury (Fig. 4.1).

Local response seen in extremity ischemia is a part of reperfusion syndrome masquerading as limb swelling which further accentuates the ongoing insult. The tissue most vulnerable to ischemia is the skeletal muscle which undergoes irreversible damage by 6 hours. Microvascular changes follow with cellular damage leading to no flow phenomenon. This is also seen in limb replantation.

Three processes play a role in no reflow phenomenon, i.e., intracellular calcium load, oxygen free radical damage, and faulty arachidonic acid metabolism.

Reactive oxygen species (ROS) plays a role in the body's defense mechanisms against pathogens as well as in tissue repair. ROS lead to apoptosis triggers. ROS

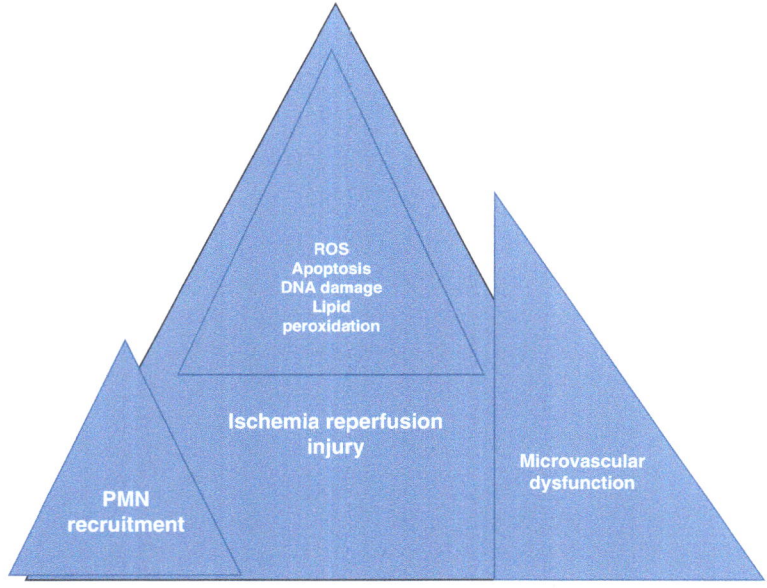

Fig. 4.1 Triangle of IRI with mediators involved

generated by neutrophils have both beneficial and harmful effects on cells. The beneficial effects of ROS include initial wound protection, PMN recruitment, tissue repair, stimulation of revascularization, and mediation of wound healing process through mediators (Fig. 4.1). However, ROS levels are controlled by intracellular antioxidants.

Microcirculatory insufficiency leads to ischemia and necrosis, macrophage activation, and the cyclic release of ROS and cytokines in ischemia phase. Reperfusion phase ie no reflow phenomenon involves endothelial and mitochondrial injury with oxidative burst of ROS.

A hyperoxic tissue environment is accompanied by more dissolved oxygen, followed by increased ROS and reactive nitrogen species (RNS) production. ROS and RNS can provoke many injurious effects on different macromolecules, including proteins, lipids, and DNA. When returning to normoxia, levels of oxygen and ROS are normalized, but the scavenger activity remains high for a prolonged period.

HBO suppresses apoptotic cell death pathways by activating the activity of mitochondria and modifying the cellular hypoxia sensor HIF-1α and its downstream pathways. Suppression of ICAM-1 expression on endothelial cells, suppression of β2-integrin expression on leukocytes leads to inhibition of leukocyte adhesion on vascular endothelial cells.

Role of Hyperbaric

HBO ameliorates the detrimental effects of IR injury by improving tissue microcirculation and hyperoxygenation. Free radical scavenging systems, specifically SOD, may also be upregulated following HBO treatment in compromised skin flaps.

HBO has also been shown to upregulate antioxidant gene expression in human endothelial cells. HBO appears to produce its beneficial effects on ischemic tissue by both decreasing production of ROS and increasing their degradation. HBO-induced inhibition of apoptosis and improvement in cellular proliferation following renal IR injury helps in delayed graft function after renal transplant. Stabilization of mitochondrial membranes decreases apoptosis and cytochrome C release. Microcirculation is improved by NO pathway (vasodilatation), reduces oedema and capillary leakage and enhances angiogenesis.HBO mediated ROS inhibit PMN adhesion to endothelial cells.

HBOT has three mechanisms of actions: increasing oxygen partial pressure, stimulating favorable vascular effects, and augmenting physical pressure. Due to the increase in arterial and capillary oxygen tension, oxygen is delivered through endothelial diffusion in order to increase oxygen tension in tissue. Hyperbaric preconditioning can be of benefit in focal cerebral ischemia, myocardial ischemia, and traumatic brain injury. These effects can only be effective if HBOT therapy is initiated within 6 hours of insult. UHMS approved indications like compromised flaps, traumatic brain injury, crush injuries, and necrotizing infections based on IRI benefit with HBOT therapy. A thesis on compromised flaps in our hospital found a beneficial role of HBOT in 19 flaps which showed good results and were salvaged. A flow chart (Fig. 4.1) explains the interplay of ischemia reperfusion injury and treatment by HBOT. The ischemia phase is characterized by decreased blood flow (low oxygen) improved by hyperoxygenation. Calcium influx leads to mitochondrial injury stabilized by HBOT by preventing apoptosis. Reperfusion phase has ROS burst nullified by therapy in the form of increase in SOD and catalase. It exerts anti inflammatory effects by decreasing release of cytokines. NO pathway explains the integrity of microcirculation by improving perfusion in no reflow phenomenon.

Discussion

Ischemia can cause reversible or irreversible cell or tissue damage and hyperbaric oxygen can significantly reduce ischemia-hypoxia injury to the brain, spinal cord, kidney, and myocardium.

HBO suppressed apoptosis, which caused inflammation after renal I/R, promoted tubular cell regeneration. HBO has protective effects against AKI caused by renal I/R through the inhibition of apoptosis [1].

There is a reduction of neutrophil adhesion to endothelial cells following treatment of chronic wound conditions reversed by HBO treatment [2].

HBO exerts antiapoptotic effects directly via the LC3II and Bcl-2 [3]. 11 studies documented an increase in TNF alpha with 9 publications showing increase in SOD with HBO proving mechanisms of cytoprotection and anti apoptotic effects to be true in role of HBO [4].

In human coronary artery endothelial cells, HBO aided the enhancement of neovascularization by altering proangiogenic RNA [5].

Hyperbaric oxygen was further found to trigger thioredoxin-mediated signaling cascades reducing ROS production [6]. HBO therapy reverses the pAkt and beta catenin apoptosis expression factors in TBI mouse model cases outlining it's beneficial role [7].

HBO treatment significantly increased the expression of Claudin-1 and E-cadherin, inhibited intestinal tissue oxidative stress as demonstrated by upregulation of superoxide dismutase and glutathione, and HBO downregulated malondialdehyde [8].

HBO decreases ischemia-reperfusion-induced neutrophil-intercellular adhesion molecule-1 (ICAM-1) adhesion by blocking CD18 polarization [9].

Hyperbaric oxygen enhances the tolerance of normothermic, microvascular flaps to prolonged secondary ischemia [10].

Ischemia perfusion injury plays an important role in stroke patients where neutrophil adhesion to the endothelium is explored as a therapeutic target with hyperbaric therapy. It has clinical implications in management of myocardial infarction, compartment syndrome, replantation, renal failure, and revascularization. Hyperbaric preconditioning does help in reducing morphologic and functional sequelae of ischemic insults.

References

1. Migita H, Yoshitake S, Tange Y, Choijookhuu N, Hishikawa Y. Hyperbaric oxygen therapy suppresses apoptosis and promotes renal tubular regeneration after renal ischaemia/reperfusion injury in rats. Nephrourol Mon. 2016;8:e34421.
2. Kendall AC, Whatmore JL, Winyard PG, Smerdon GR, Eggleton P. Hyperbaric oxygen treatment reduces neutrophil-endothelial adhesion in chronic wound conditions through S-nitrosation. Wound Repair Regen. 2013;21(6):860–8.
3. Kovacevic S, Mitovic N, Brkic P, Ivanov M, Zivotic M, Miloradovic Z, Nesovic OJ. Hyperbaric oxygenation: can it be a novel supportive method in acute kidney injury? Data obtained from experimental studies. Cells. 2024;13(13):1119.
4. Lindenmann J, Smolle C, Kamolz LP, Smolle-Juettner FM, Graier WF. Survey of molecular mechanisms of hyperbaric oxygen in tissue repair. Int J Mol Sci. 2021;22:11754.
5. Shyu K-G, Wei Wang B-W, Pan C-M, Fang W-J, Lin C-M. Hyperbaric oxygen boosts long noncoding RNA MALAT1 exosome secretion to suppress microRNA-92a expression in therapeutic angiogenesis. Int J Cardiol. 2019;274:271–8.
6. Zhen-Ni G, Xu L, Hu Q, Matei N, Yang P, Tong L-S, He Y, Guo Z, Tang J, Yang Y, et al. Hyperbaric oxygen preconditioning attenuates hemorrhagic transformation through reactive oxygen species/thioredoxin-interacting protein/nod-like receptor protein 3 pathway in hyperglycemic middle cerebral artery occlusion rats. Crit Care Med. 2016;44:e403–11.
7. He H, Li X, He Y. Hyperbaric oxygen therapy attenuates neuronal apoptosis induced by traumatic brain injury via Akt/GSK3beta/beta-catenin pathway. Neuropsychiatr Dis Treat. 2019;15:369–74.
8. Liu X, Liang F, Song W, Diao X, Zhu W, Yang J. Effect of Nrf2 signaling pathway on the improvement of intestinal epithelial barrier dysfunction by hyperbaric oxygen treatment after spinal cord injury. Cell Stress Chaperon. 2021;26:433–41.
9. Jones SR, Carpin KM, Woodward SM, et al. Hyperbaric oxygen inhibits ischemia-reperfusion-induced neutrophil CD18 polarization by a nitric oxide mechanism. Plast Reconstr Surg. 2010;126:403–11.
10. Stevens DM, Weiss DD, Koller WA, Bianchi DA Survival of normothermic microvascular flaps after prolonged secondary ischemia: effects of hyperbaric oxygen. Otolaryngol Head Neck Surg. 1996;115(4):360–4.

Chapter 5
Contraindications of Hyperbaric

Introduction

Certain risks are associated with the use of hyperbaric chambers. A monoplace chamber is designed to handle a single person whereas multiplace chambers can accommodate up to 6–20 people at a time. Every person needs to be screened before entering the chamber.

Absolute Contraindications

According to UHMS and ECHM, untreated pneumothorax is the only absolute contraindication of HBOT. Pulmonary over-pressurization may also occur as a consequence of acute and chronic pulmonary pathologies. The reactivation of latent tuberculosis exacerbates ongoing damage. If decompressed, the gas in the pleural space expands causing respiratory distress and eventually cardiac arrest. The risk factors are mechanical ventilation.

Relative Contraindications

The relative contraindications of HBOT are:

V. Mago, *Hyperbaric Medicine*, https://doi.org/10.1007/978-981-95-2644-4_5

Heart Failure

Patients with reduced left ventricular ejection fraction (<35%) causes pulmonary edema. It triggers bradycardia and electrical disturbances of the heart. Prolonged QT interval is seen in most of the patients.

Active Asthma

It leads to air trapping and triggers pulmonary barotrauma. The air cysts or blebs tend to cause pulmonary barotrauma due to air trapping.

Implanted Devices/Epidural Pain Pump

These devices pose a risk of fire or malfunction in a pressurized chamber. Epidural pain pumps can malfunction or deform due to high pressure. Transdermal patches are to be removed before entering the chamber due to risk of fire. Deep brain stimulators get deformed in a hyperbaric chamber.

Pregnancy

It poses a threat to the fetus in early pregnancy. It is given to pregnant patients with CO poisoning.

Eustachian Tube Abnormalities

Inability to equalize pressures due to previous otosclerotic surgery or infections (mastoiditis) leads to pain or barotrauma. Leaks in the inner ear lead to pressure changes.

Claustrophobia

Chamber anxiety especially in a monoplace chamber is a relative contraindication.

Optic Neuritis

History of optic neuritis in patients can lead to blindness with HBOT. Hard contact lenses are to be avoided.

Drugs and Medications

Use of doxorubicin can lead to cardio toxicity with HBOT. Cisplatin impairs wound healing. Bleomycin causes pulmonary fibrosis and should be used with caution. Disulfiram increases the risk of oxygen toxicity and so should be avoided. Mafenide leads to carbon dioxide retention. Use of cocaine or amphetamines is risky in a chamber.

Previous Surgery of Eye or Thorax

A history of eye surgery can cause expansion of gases trapped in the ocular adnexa. Thoracic surgeries pose a risk of pneumothorax.

Insulin-Dependent Diabetes and Hypoglycemia

Blood sugar levels can drop during hyperbaric sessions while treating diabetic foot ulcers. Insulin requirements decrease if HBO is administered to insulin-dependent diabetics, and hypoglycemic episodes need to be monitored.

Tuberculosis

Reactivation of latent tuberculosis can occur.

Congenital Spherocytosis

Hyperbaric leads to hemolysis as RBCs are rigid and not deformable.

Uncontrolled Epilepsy

Uncontrolled fever triggers seizures in a pressurized chamber. An air break is another risk factor. One needs to lower treatment pressures(<1.5ATA) to control seizure frequency. The frequency of seizures depends on the duration of oxygen toxicity.

Discussion

A thorough medical history evaluation is very important prior to subjecting the patient to HBOT.

HBOT is relatively contraindicated in patients with reduced left ventricular ejection fraction [1]..

HBOT is likely to trigger the reactivation of TB. High-risk patients should undergo the tuberculin skin test or interferon-gamma release assays [2].

There is a high incidence of decompression sickness in high gas loading dives that precede accelerated ascents and omitted stage decompression [3].

Any pathology in the respiratory system disqualifies a patient to dive due to risk of air trapping [4].

Continuous glucose monitoring can manage hypoglycemic episodes during hyperbaric therapy [5].

Incidence of oxygen toxicity seizures is related to increased inhaled partial pressure of oxygen and duration of treatment. The authors have proposed using the monoplace chamber for USN TT6 in selected patients to lower seizure risk [6].

The uncertainty inside the chamber, boredom, environment noise, and the hood were issues seen in chamber-related anxiety [7].

During the decompression, at the end of the hyperbaric session, the increase in gas volume related to decreasing the pressure in the chamber can induce tension pneumothorax. The risk can be minimized when pleural cavities have been drained [8].

Specific medical conditions related to the hyperbaric environment are evaluated in a strict preanesthetic checkup before placing a patient in the chamber. This avoids occurrence of untoward incidents in the chamber. The nursing officers in our hospital are fully trained to recognize the risks of the procedure based on the indication and teach Valsalva maneuver to all patients before HBOT. Early HBOT initiation can benefit many critical patients. The cancer chemotherapy drugs have to be stopped before HBOT therapy. Smoking needs to be stopped before entering a chamber. Identification of comorbidities mitigates risk of harm in hyperbaric therapy.

References

1. Schiavo S, Brenna CTA, Albertini L, Djaiani G, Marinov A, Katznelson R. Safety of hyperbaric oxygen therapy in patients with heart failure: a retrospective cohort study. PLoS One. 2024;19(2):e0293484.
2. Wang KY, Lin YS, Sy CL, Huang WC, Chen LW. Hyperbaric oxygen therapy increases the risk of tuberculosis disease. Int J Tuberc Lung Dis. 2018;22(6):637–40.
3. Clarke D, Gerard W, Norris T. Pulmonary barotrauma-induced cerebral arterial gas embolism with spontaneous recovery: commentary on the rationale for therapeutic compression. Aviat Space Environ Med. 2002;73(2):139–46.
4. Sutherland A. Contraindications to diving. SPUMS J. 1986;16(1):21–2.
5. Baines C, Vicendese D, Cooper D, McGuiness W, Miller C. Comparison of venous, capillary and interstitial blood glucose data measured during hyperbaric oxygen treatment from patients with diabetes mellitus. Diving Hyperb Med. 2021;51(3):240–7.
6. Bonnington S, Banham N, Foley K, Gawthrope I. Oxygen toxicity seizures during United States navy treatment table 6: an acceptable risk in monoplace chambers? Diving Hyperb Med. 2021;51(2):167–72.
7. Chalmers A, Mitchell C, Rosenthal M, Elliott D. An exploration of patients' memories and experiences of hyperbaric oxygen therapy in a multiplace chamber. J Clin Nurs. 2007;16(8):1454–9.
8. Kot J, Michałkiewicz M, Sićko Z. Odma opłucnowa w trakcie leczenia hiperbarycznego [Pneumothorax during hyperbaric oxygenation]. Anestezjol Intens Ter. 2008;40(1):35–8.

Chapter 6
Hyperbaric Medicine in Chronic Wounds

Introduction

Nonhealing wounds are hypoxic where normal wound healing cascade is disturbed. About 15–25% of people with diabetes will develop a foot ulcer. The chronicity of diabetic foot ulcers is due to the anatomical deformity with a disturbed plantar loading. HBOT acts as a bactericidal, stops toxin production, and promotes tissue growth to heal difficult wounds. It is thought to aid wound healing by supplying oxygen to the wound. Twenty-three percent of adults in the USA have varicose veins affecting the lower limbs. The various perforators, followed by the great saphenous vein, were the most commonly affected veins in males, slightly more common on the left side. In India, varicose veins occur in 30% of the population. Treatment incurred is a financial burden to the patient and healthcare providers. Alternate treatment modalities like hyperbaric medicine can bring a revolution in wound care by their immediate and late effects in different stages of wound healing.

Biology of Wound Healing

A healing wound passes through the amalgamation of 4 phases:

1. Hemostasis

   When a wound occurs, the first step is that blood oozes from the capillaries into the wound, releasing numerous platelets and fibrinogen. Fibrinogen activates platelets to release PDGF, TGF alpha, and VEGF. Formation of blood clots occurs once platelets come in contact with damaged extracellular matrix.

V. Mago, *Hyperbaric Medicine*, https://doi.org/10.1007/978-981-95-2644-4_6

2. Inflammation

Neutrophils enter the wounded site within 24 hours to promote phagocytosis of the foreign bodies, blood clot, and debris. The growth factors released allow monocytes to reach the site which become macrophages responsible to engulf dead neutrophils and necrotic debris. During this phase, fibroblasts become active which arise from damaged extracellular matrix.

3. Proliferation

Fibroblasts promote proliferative phase of healing which is oxygen-dependent. This phase exemplifies the role of hyperbaric therapy at cellular level, promoting collagen production by fibroblasts. The formation of granulation tissue is a by-product of fibroblasts. These fibroblasts convert into myofibroblasts along extracellular matrix, providing tensile strength to the wound. The fibroblasts secrete growth factors attracting keratinocytes into the wound, facilitating formation of new blood vessels. This process of new blood vessels network brings oxygen and other nutrients into the wound site, stimulating healing of the wound.

4. Remodeling

This phase lasts from months to years, causing collagen remodeling favoring wound contraction. The tensile strength increases from 20% in 3 weeks to about 80% in a span of 2 years.

Etiology of Chronic Wounds

A variety of causes lead to the formation of chronic wounds.

1. Diabetes.
2. Arterial insufficiency.
3. Varicose veins.
4. Pressure ulcers.
5. Neuropathic.
6. Hematological.
7. Neoplasms.
8. Trauma.

Diabetes

Diabetic foot ulcer cases are on the rise in India, the USA, and globally, posing a threat being associated with infection, amputations, and deaths. It affects 6.2% people in India and accounts for 1.6 million people in the USA. The overall incidence

Fig. 6.1 Diabetic foot
ulcer over heel with
maceration

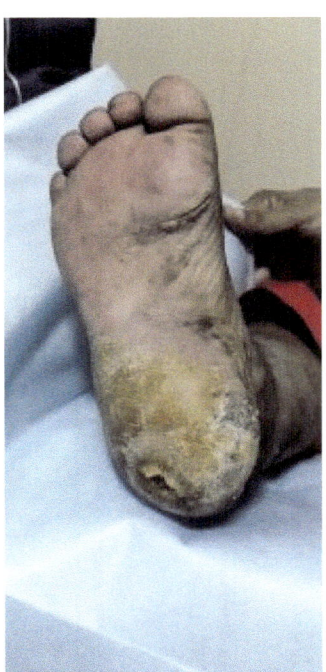

of amputation has reached 50%. Minor trivial trauma is the most common inciting factor. Elevated pressures at plantar weight-bearing areas (Fig. 6.1) lead to ulcers.

The relapse rate for these ulcers is 66%. The incidence of major amputation is 0.5–5/1000 persons with diabetes. Minor trivial trauma leads to skin breakdown. The 6 stages of diabetic foot as proposed by International diabetes conference is:

1. Stage 1—normal foot.
2. Stage 2—high risk foot.
3. Stage 3—ulcerated foot.
4. Stage 4—cellulitic foot.
5. Stage 5—necrotic foot.
6. Stage 6—foot that cannot be rescued.

Patients with type-2 diabetes are more prone for ulceration. Wagner classification is a useful tool based on the depth of wound and type of necrotic tissue. The size, area, depth, sepsis, arthropathy, and denervation (SAD) is another classification useful in research and audits. The risk factors involved are neuropathy, vasculopathy, and foot deformities. Classic neuropathic ulcers are painless punched out present on weight-bearing areas, sometimes presenting as gangrene or ulcers (Fig. 6.2).

Fig. 6.2 Post-diabetes
ulcer over right foot

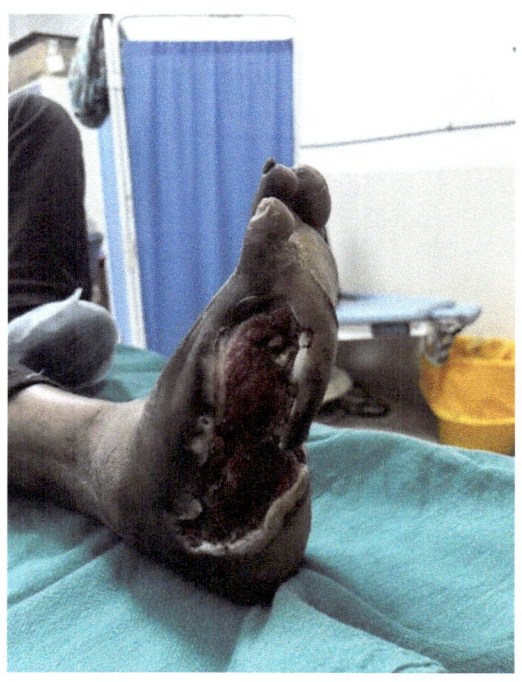

Venous Ulcer

Venous ulcers are a consequence of long-standing varicose veins seen in elderly patients and who stay on their feet for long periods. In 90% of cases, the involvement of the deep system of veins is seen. The most common site is around the ankle in the form of a shallow ulcer with pale granulation on the floor. The varicose veins are visible camouflaged by hyperpigmented dermatosclerotic skin (Fig. 6.3).

It is caused by venous reflux or obstruction. They affect 1–2% of the population.

Arterial Insufficiency

Poor circulation is a cause of peripheral arterial disease due to atherosclerosis. Reduced blood flow causes calf or thigh pain with walking. The risk factors are old age, smoking, obesity, hypertension, high cholesterol, and homocysteine levels. It affects 200 million worldwide and prevalence in India varies from 7.6% to 26.7%. The ankle brachial and duplex ultrasound are advised for its diagnosis. Rutherford classification is used to rate the walking impairment in these patients. Toe brachial index is used if ABI >1.4 in patients with arterial insufficiency. These ulcers are

Fig. 6.3 Venous ulcer over medial malleolus with hyperpigmentation

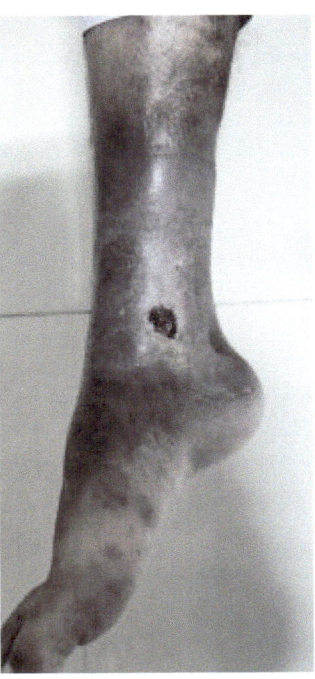

Fig. 6.4 Grade 4 pressure sore over sacrum

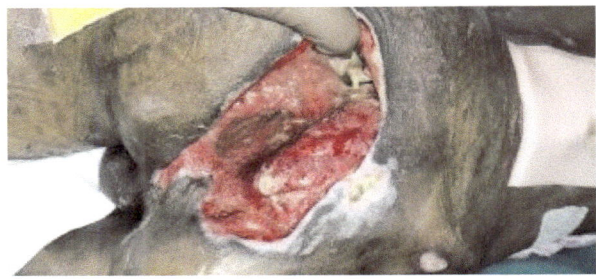

located on the lateral malleolus or distal digits. It is punched out and very painful. A Curling's ulcer is an ischemic ulcer which develops in the duodenum. These ulcers respond best to HBOT therapy.

Pressure Ulcers

Ulcers over the bony prominences due to prolonged pressure are a serious concern. Seventy percent of these bed sores are present over the sacrum, greater trochanter, and ischial tuberosity (Fig. 6.4). Predominant risk factors are poor nutrition, decreased mobility, moisture and sensory loss. The overall prevalence of bed sores in India is 7.8% and burden in ICU patients is 24.3%. The prevalence of bed sores in the USA is 2.5 million. The Covid-19 pandemic led to a resurgence of bed sore cases due to prolonged length of stay and use of multiple medical devices. Braden scale score is used as a risk assessment tool for pressure ulcers.

Neuropathic

Patients with neurological disorders develop ulcers over pressure points due to lack of sensation (Fig. 6.5). The most common site is the lower extremity secondary to toxins, amyloid, shingles, or autoimmune disorders. The etiology of these ulcers is based on anatomical, systemic, toxic, or metabolic factors. Charcot neuroarthropathy is another spectrum of neuropathic ulcerations and infections.

Hematologic

The lower leg is the most common site for sickle cell ulcers with bilateral involvement. These ulcers are common on the African continent, and in India seen on the Deccan plateau area, Kerala, Tamil Nadu, and Raipur. Vaso-occlusion is the hallmark of this disease. Severe disease is seen in children characterized by >3 bone pain crises and > 3 transfusions/year.

Fig. 6.5 Post-polio neuropathic ulcer right foot

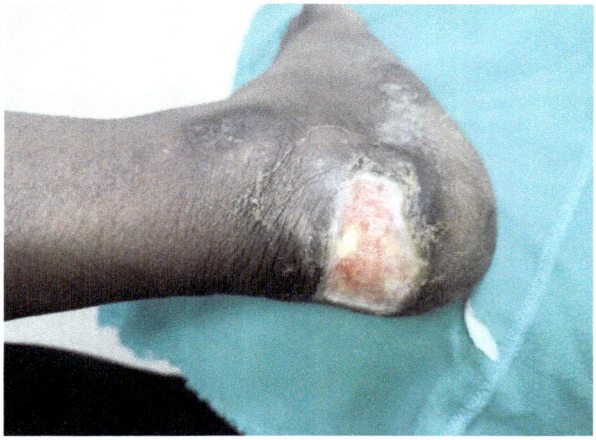

Neoplasms

Cutaneous malignancies like basal cell carcinoma or squamous cell carcinoma present with ulceration(Fig. 6.6). Marjolin's ulcer arises from burn scars. It is a highly aggressive squamous cell carcinoma involving scalp, extremities, and the gluteal region.

Trauma

Trauma is one of the foremost inciting agents to inflict formation of acute or chronic wounds. Facial lacerations can lead to wounds of varying sizes and cause disfigurement and scarring. HBOT plays an important role in various stages of progression of wounds of facial lacerations (Fig. 6.7a). The crush injury of extremities are very commonly seen in the OPD with varying degrees of ulcers and gangrenous changes (Fig. 6.7b).

Fig. 6.6 Marjolin's ulcer over right shoulder, arm, and back

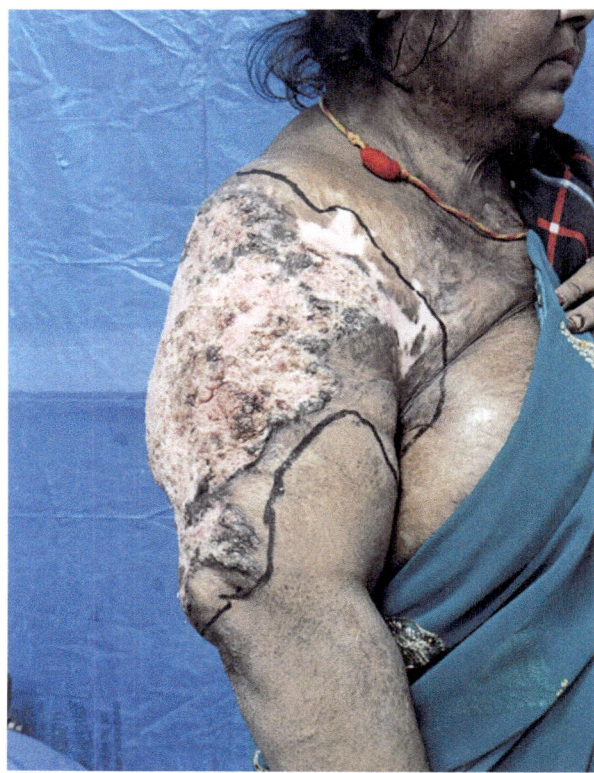

Fig. 6.7 (**a**) Post-trauma lacerations over face. (**b**) Crush injury right leg with gangrenous changes

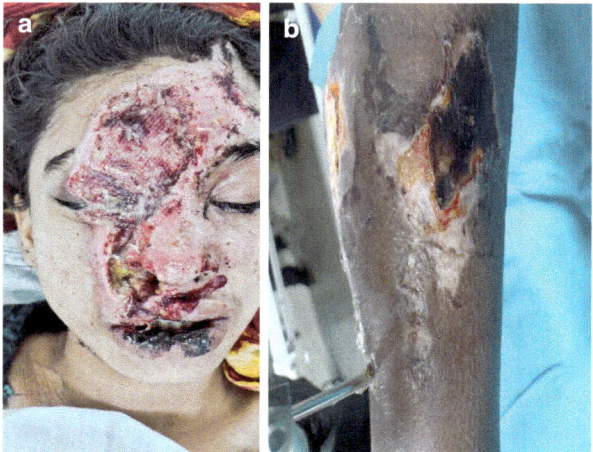

Table 6.1 Factors affecting wound healing

Local	Systemic	Immunological
Oxygenation	Stress	Adipokines
Infection	Obesity	Chemokines
Foreign body	Alcoholism	Cytokines
Venous insufficiency	Smoking	
Friction	Increased age	
Seroma formation	Malnutrition	
Pannus formation	Vitamins-A, C, E, trace elements—Zn, Cu	

Risk Factors

It can be both local or systemic causes. Table 6.1 elucidates the local and systemic factors affecting the wound healing in a chronic wound.

High altitude favors a prolonged time for wounds to heal and similar situation is felt in deep sea divers where wounds healed faster emphasizing role of oxygen in wound healing. High blood sugars can impair wound healing. Overweight individuals are at an increased risk of infection. Peripheral arterial disease predisposes to chronic ulcers and risk of amputation. Poor diet, alcoholism, and smoking retard the wound healing. Excessive pressure impedes blood flow and impairs healing, as in bed sores. Proper nutrient intake is also important for a wound to heal.

Elderly population exhibit delayed healing of wounds. Deficiency of trace elements like Zinc or Copper and Vitamins A, C, and E impairs wound healing.

Pathophysiology of Wound Healing

Chronic wounds are characterized by hypoxia, prolonged inflammation, and impaired angiogenesis. The therapeutic benefits can be derived based on gas concentrations, volume, and pressure. Increasing partial pressure of oxygen in arterial blood during HBOT improves the cellular delivery and supply of oxygen. The normal oxygen concentration of plasma at sea level is 3 mL/L. At a pressure of 3 ATM breathing 100% oxygen, the plasma oxygen concentration approaches 60 mL/LA, proper oxygen tension is also needed for a wound to heal. A wound requires a tissue oxygen tension of 20 mmHg. If oxygen tension is low, there is more necrotic debris and the immune system is deficient in overcoming it. Another effect of hyperbaric oxygen therapy is decreasing surrounding edema and increasing neovascularity in ischemic tissue. It can also be bacteriostatic and bactericidal at higher concentrations. Hyperbaric oxygen therapy neutralizes alpha exotoxins produced by bacteria such as *Clostridium*. *Table 6.2 outlines the various functions of oxygen promoting healing of wounds in relation to HBOT.* Hyperoxygenation halts the cascade of infectious progress by improving the function of neutrophilic granulocytes and reduces tissue edema. It improves red cell flexibility, thereby promoting blood flow. It reduces tissue edema by vasoconstriction. it preserves intracellular ATP and decreases lactate production. Oxygen is needed by neutrophils to release reactive oxygen species that kill bacteria. It reduces wound infection by a direct action on anaerobic bacteria.

Table 6.2 Role of oxygen in healing cascade in relation to hyperbaric therapy

Function	HBOT therapy
Fuel for cellular reactions	Adds more oxygen for neutrophils
Synthesis and cross link collagen	Promotes more cross-linking of collagen
Cofactor for nitric oxide and hydrogen peroxide	Stimulates healing by elevating oxygen tension
Cofactor for reactive oxygen species	Promotes angiogenesis
Stimulate redox switch	Adequate improved antioxidant defenses
Hyperoxygenation increases VEGF and hastens angiogenesis	Main role at high pressures
Increases fibroblasts proliferation	Augments proliferation
Keratinocytes migration accelerated	Enhances keratinocytes activity

Schedule of Hyperbaric Therapy in Wounds

A typical treatment protocol is daily exposures to 2.0–2.4 atmospheres absolute (ATA) for 90–120 min for 20–40 days. Treatments have so-called air breaks, where a patient breathes just air for 5 min once or twice through the course of a treatment. This regimen raises the pulmonary O_2 tolerance of patients with subsequent sessions. Wounds like venous ulcers need 20 sessions and HBOT leads to a dramatic relief in their pain in 80% of cases with good ulcer healing. The penumbra of the ulcer improves. The arterial ulcers have shown a lot of improvement with this modality and after ten sessions, there is a reduction in the size of the ulcer (Figs. 6.8 and 6.9). Gaped abdominal wounds respond well with improvement noted after 5 sessions.

Fig. 6.8 Arterial ulcer right leg

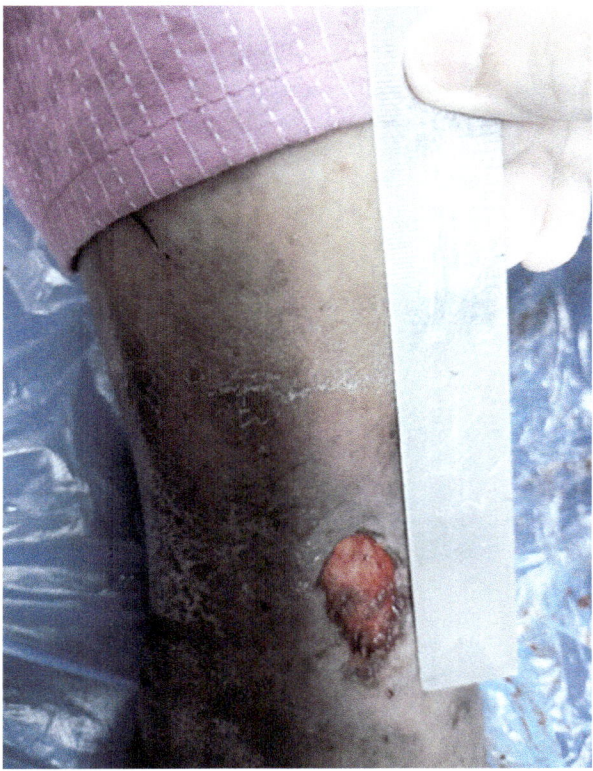

Fig. 6.9 Reduction in size
of ulcer after ten sessions

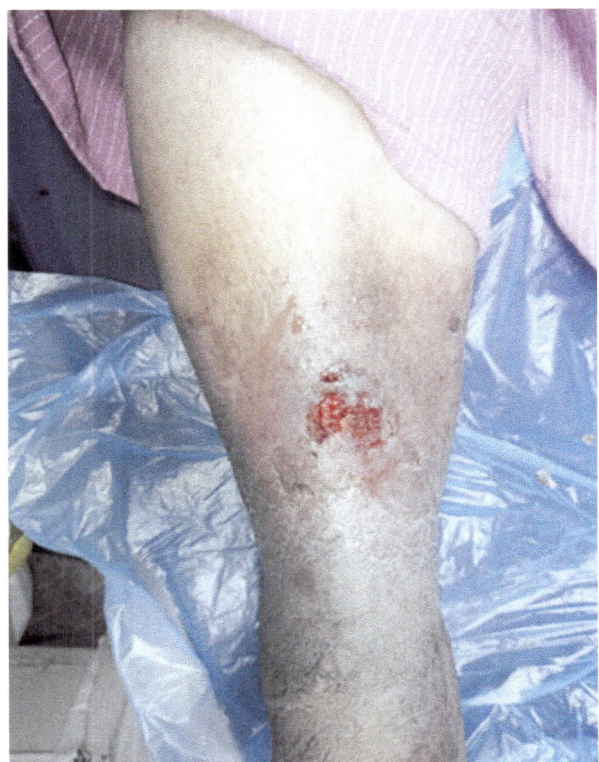

Evaluation

The response of hyperbaric to ulcer healing is checked by transcutaneous oximetry by giving an oxygen challenge justifying starting sessions in a hyperbaric chamber. It is an objective assessment of local tissue oxygenation. If a patient has values of Tc PO_2 40 mm Hg, the patient will have a good response to HBOT. If the values are between 20 and 40 mmHg, then no benefit will be derived.

Wound Healing in Diabetic Patients

A grading score by Wagner determines the treatment and types of these ulcers (Table 6.3). These ulcers can predispose to gangrene of toes, cellulitis, or abscess. The presence of infection is the most common complication. Sensory and motor neuropathy is also seen. Peripheral vasculopathy is assessed by the duplex examination. Wound debridement and amputation are done to speed up healing. Compartment syndrome is treated by fasciotomy. Sessions of HBOT are given alongside the

Table 6.3 Wagner grading

Ulcer grading	Description
Grade 0	No ulcer; foot at risk
Grade 1	Superficial ulcer
Grade 2	Deep ulcer no bony involvement
Grade 3	Abscess with bony involvement
Grade 4	Localized gangrene (fore foot)
Grade 5	Extensive gangrene whole foot

Fig. 6.10 Right diabetic foot ulcer over heel

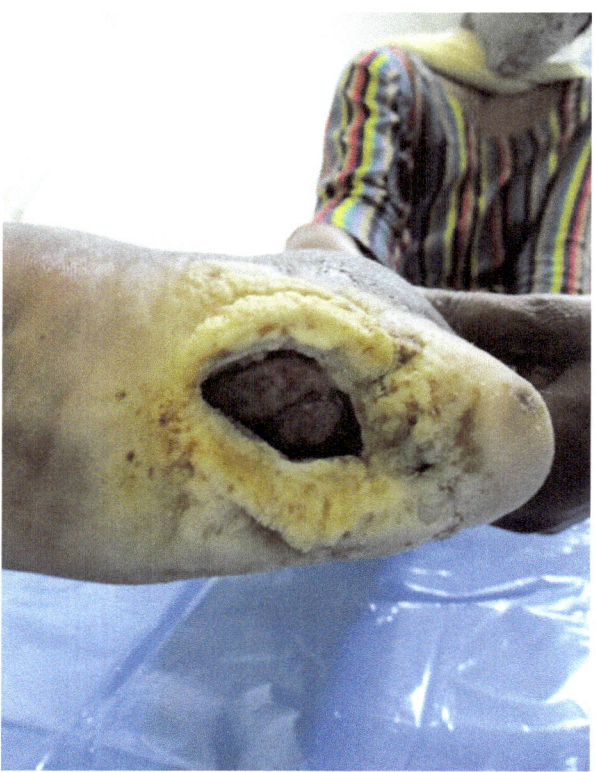

debridements to speed up healing, prepare a good wound bed and improve vascular supply. The size of ulcers decrease after ten sessions of HBOT with good wound bed and reduced tissue edema (Figs. 6.10 and 6.11).

In venous ulcers, HBOT sessions ranged from 20 to 40 with a pressure of 2.5 ATA for 90 min 5 days a week.

The stages of diabetic foot grading which respond to hyperbaric therapy are mostly from Wagner 2 to 4 based on the literature search. In our hospital, mostly Wagner grades 1–3 showed favorable response, with HBOT and simultaneous debridements.

Fig. 6.11 Reduction in size after ten HBOT sessions

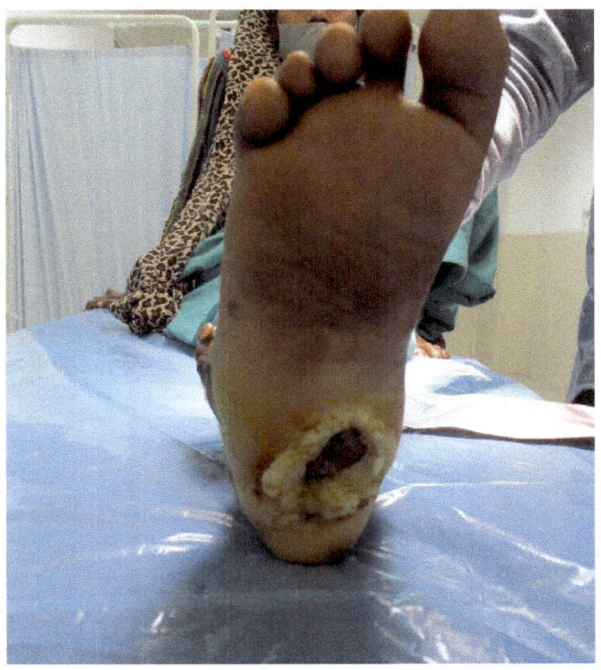

Discussion

Wound hypoxia is the major reason recalcitrant wounds do not heal. HBOT is very useful in the angiogenesis and infective control phases of wound healing.

The primary clinical outcomes (wound healing, hospital stay, complications) improved in the HBOT group [1].

Results of 7 RCTs in diabetic foot ulcers appear to suggest that this treatment results in lower costs and better outcomes than standard wound care alone [2]. The authors reported that based on findings from 118 patients HBOT helps prevent major amputations [3].

A randomized clinical trial in 2010 evaluating 94 patients with Wagner Grade 2, 3, or 4 DFUs found adjunctive HBOT facilitating healing in selected patients [4].

Zhao et al., on the basis of 9 RCTs, concluded reduction in wound size of diabetic foot ulcers [5].

A systematic review and meta-analysis of 9 clinical trials involving DFUs found HBOT improved the healing of DFUs and reduced the amputation rate [6].

Patients who received 1.5 ATA had a significant postoperative increase in the inflammatory markers soluble E-selectin, CD18, and heat shock protein 70. Neuropsychometric dysfunction was also significantly higher in HBOT patients [7].

Twenty-seven patients who had an increase in TCOM of >10 torr with oxygen inhalation at initial evaluation, then only 19 (70%) wounds healed with HBO therapy [8]. Patients with wound TcPo2 greater than 800 torr at 2.4 atm abs were noted to have a significantly greater improvement in Wound score [9]in male diabetic patients. Angiogenesis has been seen to increase after eight sessions in patients of osteoradioncrosis [10]. Eighty-one percent of all wounds were near complete healing or completely healed, in 13% of the cases the wound was stable, and in 2%, minor or major amputation had to be carried out [11].

The physiologic basis of wound healing has been elucidated in various clinical trials. HBO-exposed lymphocytes showed increase in cellular ferritin levels, whose induction prevent the generation of the DNA-damaging hydroxyl radical via Fenton reaction [12]. A systematic review found 4 level-1 trials, 3 level-2, and 3 case series on wounds supported the benefit of hyperbaric in wound healing [13].

HBO therapy mobilizes stem/progenitor cells through Nitric Oxide-(NO)dependent pathways, which may enhance ischemic limb perfusion and wound healing. Hyperoxia increased BM NO and circulating EPCs, effects inhibited by the NOS inhibitor N-nitro-l-arginine-methyl ester. Administration of SDF-1α into wounds reversed the EPC homing impairment and, with hyperoxia, synergistically enhanced EPC mobilization, homing, and wound healing [14]. This study found MDA to be significantly increased only after the first HBOT session and AOPP levels decreased after 15th session [15].

HBO triggers and upregulates the defense mechanisms against oxidative stress. Goldman found that HBOT reduces risk of amputation in the DFU population by promoting partial and full healing of problem wounds [16].

Two RCTs in this review found improved healing of ischemic ulcers after 1 year [17]. Abidia et al. advocated a decrease in the size of ulcers and cost was not a deterrent factor in its management [18]. In this study, 118 patients showed a decrease in the incidence of amputations in diabetic foot, and in venous ulcers, significant reduction in area of ulcer was seen at 6 weeks [19]. This study proposed smokers are not good candidates for hyperbaric sessions [20]. This was due to high content of carbon monoxide and carbide in the smoke. A sea-level air TcPO2 < 15 mmHg, combined with an in-chamber TcPO2 < 400 mmHg, predicts failure of hyperbaric oxygen therapy [21]. HBO2 causes cytokine downregulation and growth factor upregulation. HBO2 transiently suppresses stimulus-induced proinflammatory cytokine production and affects the liberation of TNF-alpha and endothelins [22]. HBOT administration leads to increased VEGF levels, decreased TNF-α levels, and accelerated wound healing of DFU's patients [23].

A 2012 Cochrane review gave strong evidence of ulcer healing at 6 weeks by HBOT and 5 trials confirmed its role in reducing major diabetic amputations. There is a wound size reduction of 41.8% noted at 2 weeks [24]. Transcutaneous oximetry measures the skin oxygen tension in the periphery of a wound [25]. TCOM is superior to duplex scan in calcified vessels and justifies its role after completing all sessions. This study increases tissue-level hyperoxia with hyperbaric oxygen protocols (HBO2), increasing the mobilization of Endothelial Progenitor cells from the bone marrow into peripheral blood [26]. The Wound Healing Society's clinical practice guidelines (6B1a) promulgates the role of HBOT in arterial insufficiency ulcers [27]. Full recovery was observed in 36 patients with thromboangiitis obliterans with decrease in resting pain and healing of ulcers [28]. Patients' walking distance was also increased. An RCT involving 35 patients of ischemic diabetic foot ulcer showed a decreasing trend of major amputations and increased transcutaneous oxygen tension with hyperbaric therapy [29].

After 3 months, 41.7% of chronic resistant venous leg ulcers healed completely with HBOT therapy [30].

Exposing a wound to 100% oxygen speeds up healing. HBOT improves healing rates of diabetic foot ulcers and reduces the rate of amputations. The oxygen diffusion increases in barriers like exudates, cicatrix, edema, and bone. Venous ulcers heal in 6 weeks. This therapy improves the overall quality of life of the patients.

References

1. Santema TB, Stoekenbroek RM, van Steekelenburg KC, van Hulst RA, Koelemay MJ, Ubbink DT. Economic outcomes in clinical studies assessing hyperbaric oxygen in the treatment of acute and chronic wounds. Diving Hyperb Med. 2015;45(4):228–34.
2. Health Quality Ontario. Hyperbaric oxygen therapy for the treatment of diabetic foot ulcers: a health technology assessment. Ont Health Technol Assess Ser. 2017;17(5):1–142.
3. Medical Advisory Secretariat. Hyperbaric oxygen therapy for non-healing ulcers in diabetes mellitus: an evidence-based analysis. Ont Health Technol Assess Ser. 2005;5(11):1–28.
4. Löndahl M, Katzman P, Nilsson A, et al. Hyperbaric oxygen therapy facilitates healing of chronic foot ulcers in patients with diabetes. Diabetes Care. 2010;33:998–1003.
5. Zhao D, Luo S, Xu W, et al. Efficacy and safety of hyperbaric oxygen therapy used in patients with diabetic foot: a meta-analysis of randomized clinical trials. Clin Ther. 2017;39:2088–94.
6. Golledge J, Singh TP. Systematic review and meta-analysis of clinical trials examining the effect of hyperbaric oxygen therapy in people with diabetes-related lower limb ulcers. Diabet Med. 2019;36:813–26.
7. Alex J, Laden G, Cale AR, Bennett S, Flowers K, Madden L, Gardiner E, McCollum PT, Griffin SC. Pretreatment with hyperbaric oxygen and its effect on neuropsychometric dysfunction and systemic inflammatory response after cardiopulmonary bypass: a prospective randomized double-blind trial. J Thorac Cardiovasc Surg. 2005;130(6):1623–30.
8. Grolman RE, Wilkerson DK, Taylor J, Allinson P, Zatina MA. Transcutaneous oxygen measurements predict a beneficial response to hyperbaric oxygen therapy in patients with nonhealing wounds and critical limb ischemia. Am Surg. 2001;67(11):1072–9.
9. Smith BM, Desvigne LD, Slade JB, Dooley JW, Warren DC. Transcutaneous oxygen measurements predict healing of leg wounds with hyperbaric therapy. Wound Repair Regen. 1996;4(2):224–9.
10. Marx RE, Johnson RP, Kline SN. Prevention of osteoradionecrosis: a randomized prospective clinical trial of hyperbaric oxygen versus penicillin. J Am Dent Assoc. 1985;111(1):49–54.
11. Teguh DN, Bol Raap R, Koole A, Knippenberg B, Smit C, Oomen J, van Hulst RA. Hyperbaric oxygen therapy for nonhealing wounds: treatment results of a single center. Wound Repair Regen. 2021;29(2):254–60.
12. Rothfuss A, Speit G. Investigations on the mechanism of hyperbaric oxygen (HBO)-induced adaptive protection against oxidative stress. Mutat Res. 2002;508(1–2):157–65.
13. Dauwe PB, Pulikkottil BJ, Lavery L, Stuzin JM, Rohrich RJ. Does hyperbaric oxygen therapy work in facilitating acute wound healing: a systematic review. Plast Reconstr Surg. 2014;133(2):208e–15e.

14. Gallagher KA, Liu ZJ, Xiao M, Chen H, Goldstein LJ, Buerk DG, et al. Diabetic impairments in NO-mediated endothelial progenitor cell mobilization and homing are reversed by hyperoxia and SDF-1 alpha. J Clin Invest. 2007;117:1249–59.
15. Gürdöl F, Cimşit M, Oner-Iyidoğan Y, Körpinar S, Yalçinkaya S, Koçak H. Early and late effects of hyperbaric oxygen treatment cn oxidative stress parameters in diabetic patients. Physiol Res. 2008;57(1):41–7.
16. Goldman RJ. Hyperbaric oxygen therapy for wound healing and limb salvage: a systematic review. PM&R. 2009;1(5):471–89.
17. Stoekenbroek RM, Santema TB, Legemate DA, Ubbink DT, van den Brink A, Koelemay MJ. Hyperbaric oxygen for the treatment of diabetic foot ulcers: a systematic review. Eur J Vasc Endovasc Surg. 2014;47(6):647–55.
18. Abidia A, Laden G, Kuhan G, Johnson BF, Wilkinson AR, Renwick PM, Masson EA, McCollum PT. The role of hyperbaric oxygen therapy in ischaemic diabetic lower extremity ulcers: a double-blind randomised-controlled trial. Eur J Vasc Endovasc Surg. 2003;25:513–8.
19. Kranke P, Bennett M, Roeckl-Wiedmann I, Debus S. Hyperbaric oxygen therapy for chronic wounds. Cochrane Database Syst Rev. 2004;(2):CD004123.
20. Oubre CM, Roy A, Toner C, Kalns J. Retrospective study of factors affecting non-healing of wounds during hyperbaric oxygen therapy. J Wound Care. 2007;16(6):245–50.
21. Fife CE, Buyukcakir C, Otto GH, Sheffield PJ, Warriner RA, Love TL, Mader J. The predictive value of transcutaneous oxygen tension measurement in diabetic lower extremity ulcers treated with hyperbaric oxygen therapy: a retrospective analysis of 1,144 patients. Wound Repair Regen. 2002;10(4):198–207.
22. Al-Waili NS, Butler GJ. Effects of hyperbaric oxygen on inflammatory response to wound and trauma: possible mechanism of action. ScientificWorldJournal. 2006;6:425–41.
23. Semadi NI. The role of VEGF and TNF-alpha on epithelialization of diabetic foot ulcers after hyperbaric oxygen therapy. Open Access Maced J Med Sci. 2019;7(19):3177–83.
24. Washington State Health Care Authority Health Technology Assessment Program (WA HTA) (2013) Hyperbaric oxygen therapy (HBOT) for tissue damage, including wound care and treatment of central nervous system (CNS) conditions. Olympia: WA HTA
25. Uzun G, Yildiz S, Aktas S. Hyperbaric oxygen therapy in the management of nonhealing wounds in patients with critical limb ischemia. Therapy. 2008;5:99–108.
26. Gallagher KA, Goldstein LJ, Thom SR, Velazquez OC. Hyperbaric oxygen and bone marrow–derived endothelial progenitor cells in diabetic wound healing. Vascular. 2006;14(6):328–37.
27. Shah J. Hyperbaric oxygen therapy. J Am Col Certif Wound Spec. 2010;2(1):9–13.
28. Hemsinli D, Kaplan ST, Kaplan S, Yildirim F. Hyperbaric oxygen therapy in the treatment of Fontaine stage IV Thromboangiitis obliterans. Int J Low Extrem Wounds. 2016;15(4):366–70.
29. Faglia E, Favales F, Aldeghi A, et al. Adjunctive systemic hyperbaric oxygen therapy in treatment of severe prevalently ischemic diabetic foot ulcer. Diabetes Care. 1996;19:1338–43.
30. Elsharnoby AM, El-Barbary AH, Eldeeb AE, Hassan HA. Resistant chronic venous leg ulcers: effect of adjuvant systemic hyperbaric oxygen therapy versus venous intervention alone. Int J Low Extrem Wounds. 2022;

Chapter 7
Hyperbaric in Chronic Osteomyelitis

Introduction

Osteomyelitis is infection of the bone or marrow caused by infection. It is known as the "great pretender." In hyperbaric therapy, class 2 recommendation is given for refractory osteomyelitis. Long-standing infections in bone are also a leading cause of chronic ulcers of long duration. HBO is recommended in chronic refractory osteomyelitis defined as osteomyelitis lesions persisting more than 6 weeks after adequate antibiotic treatment and at least one surgery. This is seen in 21.8 cases per 100,000 person years. It is more common in males with a high prevalence in diabetes and peripheral arterial insufficiency. It is a common disease among the poor in rural India. The crush injuries of the extremities involve damage to multiple structures within the hand or lower limbs, loss of tissue, devascularization, and possibly osteomyelitis. The most common cause is postoperative infection of open fractures.

Etiology

The bone becomes a nidus of infection from trauma, ischemia, or presence of foreign bodies (Fig. 7.1). *Staph aureus* is the most common pathogen invading bones due to adhesins, leading to chronicity, invasiveness, and hematogenous spread. It survives intracellularly by linking to osteoblasts. One essential virulence factor is leukotoxin, which leads to neutrophil lysis, apoptosis, and tissue necrosis. The osteomyelitis involving sternum, spine, or skull carries a poor prognosis. Patients with Wagner grade 3 diabetic foot ulcers harbinger a nidus of osteomyelitis within the dead bone. Acute cases present with initial episodes of osteomyelitis, and chronic cases are recurrence of acute cases with sequestra or bony necrosis.

Atypical mycobacteria and fungi can lead to osteoarticular infections.

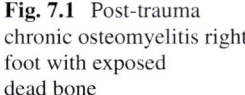

Fig. 7.1 Post-trauma
chronic osteomyelitis right
foot with exposed
dead bone

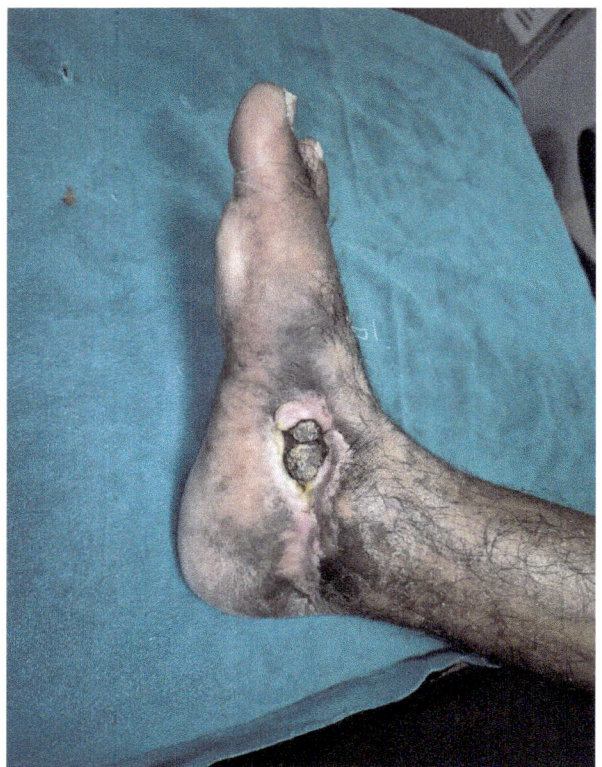

Pathology

Three factors perpetrate the occurrence of osteomyelitis in any kind of trauma.
These are:

1. Degree of tissue injury—The size and depth of wound over the extremities
   decides exposure and contamination by various bacteria.
2. Bacterium—Based on the number, strain, virulence, and reproduction rate of
   organisms, it decides level of contamination of the fracture sites. The organism
   varies with age of the patient (Table 7.1).
3. Host defense—The immunologic status, nutrition, and comorbid conditions
   accentuate the insult. The microorganisms also vary depending on the systemic
   disease, i.e., salmonella in sickle cell disease, Pseudomonas in IV drug users and
   Bartonella in HIV patients.

Table 7.1 Organism involved with corresponding age

Age of patient	Organism involved
Newborn	*Staph aureus*, *Enterobacter*
Children, adolescents	*Staph aureus*, *Streptococcus*, *H influenzae*
Adult	*Staph aureus*, occasional *Strepto* or *Enterobacter*

High energy trauma exposes bone and leads to severe tissue damage. Lack of adequate fixation of exposed fractures compounds the bacterial load and aggravates peri-osseous vascular injury. Osteonecrosis sets in with necrotic debris acting as a focus for growth of bacteria. This potentiates spread of infection in bone and extraosseous sites. The infection in dead necrotic bone leads to refractory osteomyelitis.

Staphylococcus aureus is the most common bacterium isolated in osteomyelitis, especially in posttraumatic cases. This organism promotes osteoclast production, enhancing bone destruction and osteoblast apoptosis. The leucocidin produced by *Staph aureus* promotes release of inflammatory mediators which cause massive tissue destruction. The invasion and persistence of *Staph aureus* is seen in submicron channels of cortical bone. The resistance mechanisms adopted by *Staph aureus* helps it to evade host immune treatment and antibiotics treatment. It produces toxins like alpha hemolysin (osteoblast death), canonical coagulase (inhibits osteoblast function), and leucocidin (persistence of infection). Extracellular DNA released from *Staph aureus* leads to adherence and accumulation of biofilms. These biofilms allow the bacteria to persist and reinfect.

Brodie abscess formation ensues due to ongoing tissue destruction and bone marrow infarction. The pus penetrates the Haversian canals with involvement of the periosteum destroying cortical bone. Extraosseous involvement leads to chronic ulcers and sinus formation. Local injury, hypoxia, and acidosis mediates a systemic inflammatory response syndrome or sepsis.

Modes of Bone Infection

Certain predisposing factors are important in progression and spread of bone infection via endogenous or exogenous routes (Table 7.1). Sites of involvement can be long bones of the leg, femur, sternum and jaw. The organisms responsible for osteomyelitis can take origin from hematogenous spread or contiguous mode. It can be either hematogenous or contiguous.

Hematogenous Osteomyelitis

It is monomicrobial, with no previous risk factors. It can arise from preexisting infections in the body. It represents 20% of the cases mainly found in children. Clavicular osteomyelitis occurs by hematogenous spread following head and neck surgery.

Contiguous Spread

This affects adults and is polymicrobial. It follows trauma, surgery, or surrounding infections. Most of these cases are due to trauma. Those with infections in the body are due to diabetes. Diabetic foot ulcers have a nidus of infection in their bones.

Clinical Presentation and Evaluation

Patients of chronic osteomyelitis can present with swelling, pain, or erythema in affected site and often with chronic ulcers or sinuses. Patient can limp or present with abnormal gait. Physical examination involves finding a nidus of infection with sensory evaluation and rule out peripheral vascular disease. The probe to bone test is a valuable screening tool in examination. Digital osteomyelitis is common in diabetic patients. The various risk factors and sites involved in the spread of osteomyelitis is tabulated in Table 7.2. The samples are taken from bone, blood, or wound aspirates for culture and sensitivity.

A draining sinus tract can also be a common presentation. Sometimes a patient can present with exposed dead bone (sequestrum as in Fig. 7.1). Bony X-rays of involved sites can show bone lucency, sclerotic rim, osteopenia, or lysis around embedded hardware. Figure 7.2 shows X-ray findings involving dead sclerotic bone with lytic lesions. A sequestrum is a dead bone often a nidus of infection. Involucrum

Table 7.2 Sites and risk factors for osteomyelitis

Risk factors	Site of involvement
Recent trauma or surgery	Extremities
IV drug abuse	Medial or lateral clavicle
Poor vascular supply	Foot, digits
Systemic diseases	Skull base, odontoid peg
Peripheral neuropathy	Foot, decubitus ulcers
Malignancy	
Smoking or alcohol	
Renal or liver failure	Spine and ribs

Fig. 7.2 X-ray right foot
showing osteomyelitis
involving dead sclerotic
bone with lytic lesions

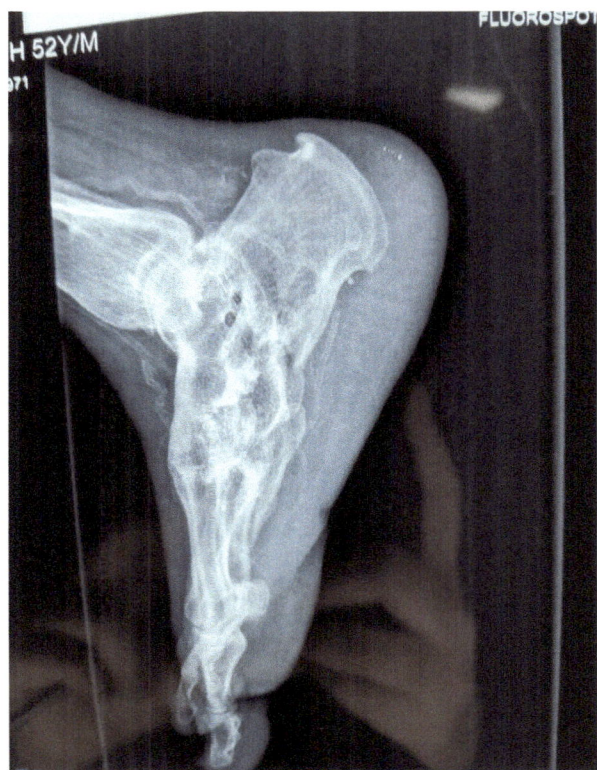

is formation of new bone around necrotic tissue. Brodie's abscess is a type of intraosseous abscess following osteomyelitis which affects the growth plate of the bone. An MRI or CT scan assists in the diagnosis and surgical planning. RI is best in early stages of osteomyelitis. A technetium bone scan or gallium scan is done when X-rays are normal. A bone culture is gold standard for starting organism-based antibiotic therapy.

Benefits of Hyperbaric

Leukocyte mediated killing of gram positive and negative organisms is mediated by hyperoxygenation. HBOT potentiates the penetration of aminoglycoside and imipenem antibiotics in infected bone. HBOT suppresses anaerobic infections. It improves vascularity and potentiates phagocytosis.

It enhances osteogenesis by improving osteoclast function. The osteoclast enhancement triggers bone debridement and prevents spread of local infections. It is effective in reducing tissue edema, intracompartment pressures, and reduce infections. It enhances bone and soft tissue healing in ischemic tissues.

Classification-Based Treatment

Cierny and Mader classification is used as a guide to demarcate which patients will benefit with HBOT therapy. Cierny Mader's anatomic staging and host status is useful for management (Table 7.3) which is based on the site of involvement and bony destruction. Table 7.4 outlines the physiologic classification based on patient's own condition. This staging system helps in adopting debridement strategies, dead space management, and antibiotic administration.

Stages 3 and 4 are best managed with HBOT combined with surgical debridement and antibiotics. Stage 3 patients need extensive debridement and excision of necrotic bone. A significant dead space is created which needs muscle flap or fasciocutaneous flap or free flap cover to obliterate it.

Stage 4 involves circumferential segment of whole bone which must be removed.

Class A hosts are normal patients. A class B has local compromised tissue. Many systemic diseases alter the ability of the body to fight infection. Smoking, alcohol, and steroids lower the immune status predisposing to infections. Class C host is a poor surgical candidate.

Dose of HBO

Timely and correct diagnosis and treatment are necessary for good results with hyperbaric oxygen therapy. Our institution adopts a protocol of giving 10 preoperative sessions of 2–2.4 ATA HBOT once a day 5 days a week. This is followed by definitive management of debridement, saucerization with flap cover, depending upon indication and further 10 postoperative sessions of HBOT (Figs. 7.3 and 7.4).

Table 7.3 Anatomic staging of osteomyelitis

Stage 1	Medullary
Stage 2	Superficial disease
Stage 3	Localized spread
Stage 4	Diffuse disease

Table 7.4 Physiologic classification

A host	Normal
B host	Systemic compromise (Bs), local (Bl), both (Bls)
C host	Treatment worse than disease

Fig. 7.3 Saucerization and debridement of dead bone in chronic osteomyelitis upper one third right tibia

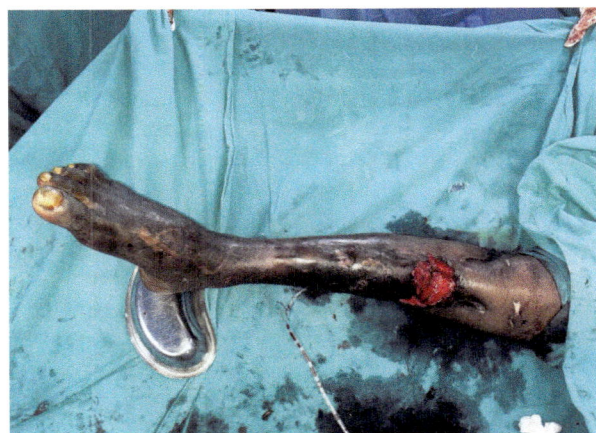

Fig. 7.4 Coverage of bone defect upper one third tibia with gastrocnemius flap and skin grafting

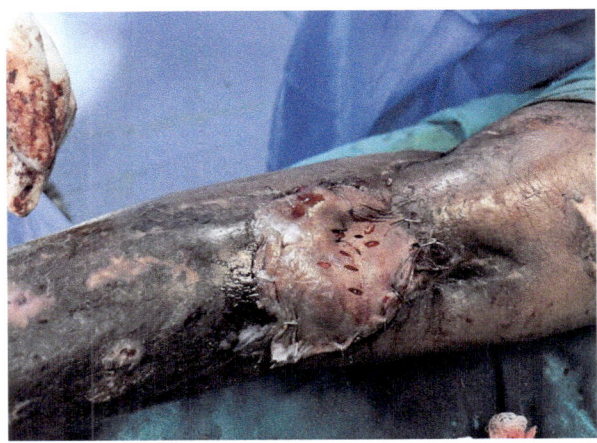

This gives good results in cases treated in our hospital and till date no recurrences have been seen. The sequestrectomy performed for osteomyelitis removes dead bone and nidus of biofilms formation. Further debridement improves the bone stock and HBOT prevents recurrence of infections. High levels of tissue oxygen penetrate bone and avascular areas with promotion of angiogenesis and new bone formation. The impregnation of aminoglycoside and imipenem antibiotics in the form of beads in cavities is potentiated by HBOT (Fig. 7.5).

Fig. 7.5 Impregnation of
antibiotic beads in
osteomyelitis cavity
Right leg

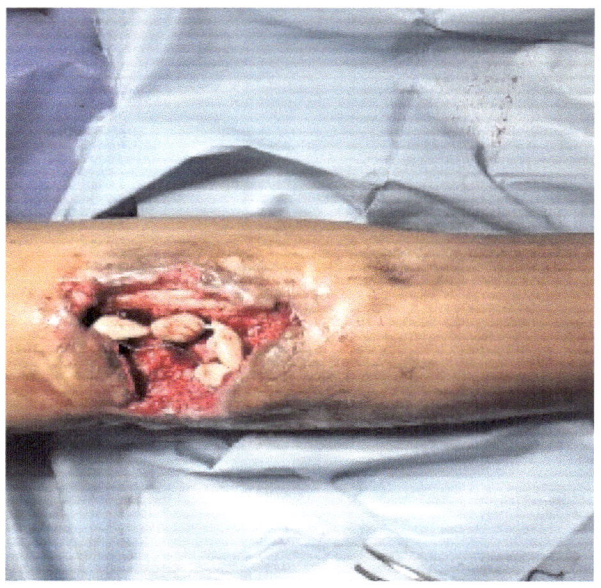

Discussion

Hyperbaric oxygen is effective in management of chronic refractory osteomyelitis once other modalities fail or patient has recurrence.

MRI diagnosed *Staph aureus* pyomyositis was treated with antibiotics and hyperbaric oxygen therapy [1].Out of the 80 patients with chronic osteomyelitis, 68 were free of infection after hyperbaric therapy over a mean follow-up of 36 months [2].

Hart has recommended an HBO dose of 2–2.4 ATA 5–7 days per week, for 90–120 minutes in osteomyelitis with therapeutic benefits [3]. In this study, six patients of chronic osteomyelitis responded to hyperbaric and saw good healing of all critical grafts with HBO [4]. HBOT acts as a bactericidal/bacteriostatic agent against anerobic bacteria by increasing the formation of free oxygen radicals. HBOT restores the bacterial-killing capacity of leukocytes in hypoxic wounds by increasing tissue oxygen tensions [5].

Staphylococcus aureus was the isolated pathogen in 12 (60%) of the 20 cohort and in 4 (20%) of the 20 case studies. Adjuvant hyperbaric oxygen was effective in 16 (80%) of the 20 cohort and 19 (95%) of the 20 case studies [6]. Forty patients of refractory osteomyelitis were treated with hyperbaric combined with surgery and antibiotics with 15% recurrence rate [7]. Diabetic foot ulcers with refractory osteomyelitis respond well with adjunct hyperbaric therapy [8]. Hyperbaric oxygen therapy enabled infection cure in 5 of 6 patients with spinal osteomyelitis complicated by medical comorbidities or the failure of primary therapy [9]. The patients who completed HBO treatment had 7.7 times the odds of experiencing refractory osteomyelitis improvement [10]. Seven out of 13 patients of osteomyelitis of the mandible in group 1 were relapse-free after performing 40 hyperbaric oxygen therapies [11], Forty-four patients manifesting chronic osteomyelitis were treated in a monoplace hyperbaric oxygen (HBO) chamber, in addition to receiving antibiotic and surgical treatment. HBO was found useful as an adjunct to help resolve the bone infection and encourage wound healing [12].

The purpose of this case study was to reflect a vasculopathic patient, poorly fit for surgical intervention with refractory osteomyelitis, had benefitted from early HBO as an adjunct to standard treatment [13].

All patients of bacterial spinal osteomyelitis remained symptom- and infection-free over the subsequent follow-up period with HBOT. Two patients had primary spinal osteomyelitis that had recurred despite a full course of appropriate antimicrobial therapy. Infection control was achieved after HBO therapy in 1 patient. The mean follow-up period for the study group was 2.9 years [14].

Complete eradication of infection in chronic refractory osteomyelitis of the femur with no recurrence of infection was noted in 12 of the 13 patients with HBO. One patient failed to respond to the treatment. The success rate of the treatment regimen was 92% [15].

HBO is a specific therapeutic measure for treatment of chronic refractory osteomyelitis combined with different modalities and sites involved. It resolves bone infection and improves wound healing. Adjuvant HBO is successful in the treatment of patients with chronic recurrent osteomyelitis of the mandible.

It is beneficial in patients of relapsing spinal osteomyelitis where standard therapy has failed. Hyperbaric oxygen (HBO) is a treatment modality that enhances blood perfusion to and improves innate immunity at the site of injury. Proper patient selection and treatment strategy based on staging gives consistent results with hyperbaric therapy.

References

1. Felwick R, Farrar M, Parry S. Idiopathic sternoclavicular osteomyelitis masquerading as a pyomyositis medically managed with antibiotics and hyperbaric oxygen. Shoulder Elbow. 2017;2(2):107–10.
2. Menekse S. Outcome of chronic foot osteomyelitis treated with hyperbaric oxygen: an observational study. Int J Low Extrem Wounds. 2023;23(1):80–5.
3. Hart BB. Hyperbaric oxygen for refractory osteomyelitis. Undersea Hyperb Med. 2021;48(3):297–321.
4. Jamil MU, Eckardt A, Franko W. Hyperbare Sauerstofftherapie. Klinische Anwendung in der Behandlung von osteomyelitis, Osteoradionekrose und der Wiederherstellungschirurgie des vorbestrahlten Unterkiefers [hyperbaric oxygen therapy. Clinical use in treatment of osteomyelitis, osteoradionecrosis and reconstructive surgery of the irradiated mandible]. Mund Kiefer Gesichtschir. 2000;4(5):320–3.
5. Cimşit M, Uzun G, Yildiz S. Hyperbaric oxygen therapy as an anti-infective agent. Expert Rev Anti-Infect Ther. 2009;7(8):1015–26.

6. Savvidou OD, Kaspiris A, Bolia IK, Chloros GD, Goumenos SD, Papagelopoulos PJ, Tsiodras S. Effectiveness of hyperbaric oxygen therapy for the management of chronic osteomyelitis: a systematic review of the literature. Orthopedics. 2018;41(4):193–9.
7. Morrey BF, Dunn JM, Heimbach RD, Davis J. Hyperbaric oxygen and chronic osteomyelitis. Clin Orthop Relat Res. 1979;144:121–7.
8. Unger HD, Lucca M. The role of hyperbaric oxygen therapy in the treatment of diabetic foot ulcers and refractory osteomyelitis. Clin Podiatr Med Surg. 1990;7(3):483–92.
9. Ahmed R, Severson MA, Traynelis VC. Role of hyperbaric oxygen therapy in the treatment of bacterial spinal osteomyelitis. J Neurosurg Spine. 2009;10(1):16–20.
10. Jackson JB 3rd, Bakaes Y, Jacques B, Gauthier C, Mills WL Jr, Nguyen K, Gonzalez T, Cone DL. Adjunctive hyperbaric oxygen therapy for patients with chronic refractory osteomyelitis: a report of treatment outcomes and risk factors for treatment failure. Adv Skin Wound Care. 2025;38(1):40–5.
11. Handschel J, Brüssermann S, Depprich R, Ommerborn M, Naujoks C, Kübler NR, Meyer U. Hyperbare Sauerstofftherapie bei Unterkiefer-osteomyelitis [evaluation of hyperbaric oxygen therapy in treatment of patients with osteomyelitis of the mandible]. Mund Kiefer Gesichtschir. 2007;11(5):285–90.
12. Eltorai I, Hart GB, Strauss MB. Osteomyelitis in the spinal cord injured: a review and a preliminary report on the use of hyperbaric oxygen therapy. Paraplegia. 1984;22(1):17–24.
13. Delasotta LA, Hanflik A, Bicking G, Mannella WJ. Hyperbaric oxygen for osteomyelitis in a compromised host. Open Orthop J. 2013;7:114–7.
14. Ahmed R, Severson MA III, Traynelis VC. Role of hyperbaric oxygen therapy in the treatment of bacterial spinal osteomyelitis. J Neurosurg Spine. 2009;10(1):16–20.
15. Chen CE, Ko JY, Fu TH, Wang CJ. Results of chronic osteomyelitis of the femur treated with hyperbaric oxygen: a preliminary report. Chang Gung Med J. 2004;27(2):91–7.

Chapter 8
Hyperbaric Medicine in Infertility

Introduction

Infertility is on the rise in urban settings due to late marriages and late onset of child births. Approximately 1 in 6 persons are affected by infertility and prevalence has increased from 3.5% to 16.7% in developed nations. In the USA, 7.4% of women and men are infertile. Highest rate of male infertility is seen in Asia. The male is solely responsible in 20% of cases. Smoking has deleterious effects on infertility issues of women and tend to cause early menopause. High alcohol consumption displays a U shaped relationship. The lean thin patients or obese women are more prone for infertility. As men age, testosterone levels decline and infertility rises. Men can have more DNA damage after 40 years with a decline in motility and viability of sperms. Increasing maternal and paternal age is also responsible for more infertility cases. Spontaneous abortion and implantation loss is common in old age. Oxidative stress leads to sperm dysfunction. Consuming trans fats and meat also contributes to infertility. Oocyte depletion, pelvic inflammatory disease and painful menstrual cycles are additional risk factors. Table 8.1 outlines the various modifiable lifestyle factors and diseases related to female infertility.

South India has more women affected by infertility due to late marriage, unhealthy food, and obesity. Hyperbaric as a modality works by improving endometrial receptivity by improving oxygenation.

Spermatogenesis in males is affected by temperature, environment, and toxins. Besides motor loss, spinal cord injured patients suffer from erectile and ejaculatory dysfunctions and spermatogenesis deficiencies which improve with HBOT. Lead toxicity and ionizing radiation are also responsible for infertility. The blockages that prevent delivery of sperms is another factor. Covid-19 also showed a reduction in sperm count. Varicoceles also contribute to male infertility due to low sperm count and impaired Leydig cell function. Methyl mercury in fish and shellfish consumption leads to infertility.

V. Mago, *Hyperbaric Medicine*, https://doi.org/10.1007/978-981-95-2644-4_8

Table 8.1 Risk Factors
leading to female infertility

Modifiable lifestyle factors	Diseases
Obesity	PCOD
Underweight	Endometriosis
Smoking	Thyrotoxicosis
Alcohol	Hyperprolactinemia
Drugs	
Toxins	

Table 8.2 Lifestyle factors and conditions affecting male infertility

Lifestyle factors	Other factors
Smoking	Varicocele, vasectomy, cryptorchidism
Alcohol	Increased age
Drug	Hypogonadism
Obesity	Congenital disorders
Toxins, pesticides	Endocrine
Heat exposure, i.e., saunas	Genetic

Endometriosis leads to defective oocytes with low implantation potential. The low metabolism in the uterus or ovaries is another factor responsible for delayed implantation. BOT can potentiate this metabolism at cellular level. A thin endometrium is characterized by high uterine blood flow impedance and poor vascular development, which further results in poor endometrial growth. Prolactinemia causes luteal phase defects in infertility. Stages 3 and 4 of endometriosis distort pelvic anatomy, obstructing motility of sperms in the fallopian tubes. Greatest risk of infertility is by chlamydia. Congenital uterine anomalies and submucosal fibroids lead to infertility by causing pregnancy losses. Decreased ovarian reserve function is an early sign of ovarian failure.

Table 8.2 illustrates the various lifestyle factors and conditions affecting male infertility.

Evaluation of Infertility

Evaluation starts with a complete sexual history and physical examination of the infertile couple. The female factors for infertility can be evaluated by vital signs and general evaluation is done followed by examination of the breasts(galactorrhea). The signs of androgen excess are noted. Uterine enlargement or pelvic masses are ruled out. The assessment of ovarian function, uterine cavity, and fallopian tubes is done. Levels of AMH indicate ovarian function (<0.5 ng/ml indicates poor reserve).

In males, one must look for undescended testicle or varicocele and signs of endocrinopathy. Endocrine panel includes LH and FSH. Semen analysis is done after 3 days of abstinence. Scrotal ultrasound is useful to diagnose varicocele or absent vas or rule out testicular pathology. A testicular biopsy is needed to rule out spermatogenic failure.

Role of Hyperbaric in Infertility

HBOT is found beneficial in cases where testicular circulation is impaired, or ischemia-reperfusion injury has developed. It leads to increased energy production by sperms.

HBOT therapy promotes healthy eggs, viable sperms, and embryo development. It stimulates angiogenesis leading to an increase in VEGF levels.

The ongoing trial in our hospital involving 11 patients has shown encouraging results in patients with infertility with increased ovarian follicles and increased endometrial thickness seen after fifth cycle of HBOT as exemplified by improved AMH levels and subendometrial flow on Doppler. The mechanism involves improvement of ATP synthesis in mitochondria of sperms. It also reduces testicular ischemia perfusion damage.

It potentiates the thin endometrium for embryo implantation in IVF procedures. The application of mild hyperbaric oxygen offers sufficient oxygen in the plasma to meet the high demand for proliferative endometrium. It can especially restore normoxia in patients with scarred or thin endometrium.

Dose of HBO in Infertility

The HBOT group receives daily HBOT for at least 10 days during the proliferative phase, at a target pressure of 2.4 atm absolute (ATA) for 90 min total treatment time.

The endometrial pattern was classified as pattern A (a triple-line pattern), B (an intermediate isoechogenic pattern), or C (a homogenous hyperechogenic pattern). Endometrial thickness monitoring in relation to the standard cycle is a crucial step during fertility treatment, and it can be easily measured by transvaginal ultrasound.

It shows increased systolic flow in preovulatory phase as compared with the follicular ovary. Oocytes retrieved from follicles with good blood flow show better implantation rates.

Discussion

Angiogenesis is crucial for oocyte quality, follicular development, and early embryo development.

The authors found an increased mean sperm count of the patients subjected to HBOT. Their pre HBOT sperm count was 8.4 ± 11.1 mil/mL, while it was found to be 15.7 ± 15.0 mil/mL after HBOT [1]. Animal studies in rats found more viable sperms in HBOT treated spinal cord injury-related infertility [2]. Varicocelectomy with HBO can more effectively regulate reproductive hormone, improve the semen quality, SPA index, and pregnancy rate [3].

Sperm viability was two times greater in the HBOT group when compared with the control group 28 days after the injury [4].

The authors reported high ovarian stimulation parameters, embryo implantation, and pregnancy rates in five patients who received HBOT [5]. Pregnancy occurred after tenth or 11th cycle. Exposure to mild hyperbaric oxygen at 1266 kPa with 36% oxygen is effective for improved outcomes of infertility treatment. Liu has shown promising results of improving premature ovarian failure with HBOT [6]. The Anti-Mullerian Hormone (AMH) serum level would be a good marker of ovarian reserve and a predictor of response to stimulation. This study showed that hyperbaric oxygen sessions can increase serum AMH levels, with a significant increase of 116% in one case [7].

The authors showed HBOT given prior to endometrium transformation contributes to increased endometrial thickness and facilitates blastocyst implantation in patients with resistant thin endometrium during FET treatments [8]. The therapy was given on 5th day of menstrual cycle in a multiplace chamber at 2.3ATA with excellent response in endometrium shown on folliculometry [9].

HBO treatment caused a significant decrease in the mean level of sperm DNA fragmentation and ongoing pregnancy after IVF occurred in 63.3% (38/60) of sexual partners of the treatment group [10].

The oxygen used as a drug in HBOT may lead to better outcome of pregnancy by improving endometrial receptivity. Increased spermatogenesis is achieved 2 months after therapy. It also leads to good effects on DNA integrity of the sperms. Early treatment with HBOT leads to better ovarian follicles for treatment. It improves ovarian function by improving oxygen storage capacity of ovarian tissue.

References

1. Özgök Kangal K, Özgök Y. Assisted reproductive treatments with hyperbaric oxygen therapy in male infertility. Turk J Urol. 2021;47(2):98–105.
2. Falavigna A, Silva PG, Conzatti LP, Corbellini LM, Cagliari CS, Pasqualotto FF. Sperm viability after spinal cord injury using hyperbaric therapy. World Neurosurg. 2018;113:e232–8.
3. Zheng RQ, Wang XS, Wang PT. Effect of varicocelectomy with hyperbaric oxygenation in treating infertile patients with varicocele. Zhonghua Nan Ke Xue. 2006;12(1):46–9.
4. Falavigna A, da Silva PG, Conzatti LP, et al. Avoiding infertility after spinal cord injury by hyperbaric oxygenation therapy. Global Spine J. 2017;5(1):s-0035-1554319.
5. Van Voorhis BJ, Greensmith JE, Dokras A, Sparks AE, Simmons ST, Syrop CH. Hyperbaric oxygen and ovarian follicular stimulation for in vitro fertilization: a pilot study. Fertil Steril. 2005;83(1):226–8.
6. Liu JY. Clinical observation of 29 cases of premature ovarian failure treated with hyperbaric oxygen. Chin J Nautical Med Hyperb Med. 2020;27(4):510–2.
7. Pineda JF, Ortiz CG, Moguel Gde J, Lopez CR, Alcocer HM, Velasco ST. Improvement in serum anti-müllerian hormone levels in infertile patients after hyperbaric oxygen (preliminary results). JBRA Assist Reprod. 2015;19(2):87–70.
8. Chen J, Huang F, Fu J, Zhao J, Li J, Peng Z, Zhao J, Xu B, Li S, Zhang Q, Liang S, Li Y. Hyperbaric oxygen therapy: a possible choice for patients with resistant thin endometrium during frozen embryo transfer treatments. Reprod Biol Endocrinol. 2023;21(1):80.
9. Mitrović A, Brkić P, Nikolić B, Dragojević S, Zaric O, Ljubić A, Jovanović T. Hyperbaric oxygen and in vitro fertilisation. Aust N Z J Obstet Gynaecol. 2006;46(5):456–7.
10. Metelev AY, Bogdanov AB, Ivkinl EV, Mitrokhin AA, Vodneva MM, Veliev EI. Hyperbaric oxygen therapy in the treatment of male infertility associated with increased sperm DNA fragmentation and reactive oxygen species in semen. Urologiia. 2015;5:74–6.

Chapter 9
Venous and Arterial Gas Embolism

Introduction

In the emergency, arterial gas embolism is seen as life threatening catastrophe with obstruction of the arterioles and venules leading to ischemia of the vital organs. Medical interventions can lead to venous embolism causing obstruction of pulmonary vasculature and cardiac chambers. HBOT is beneficial in cases of venous embolism by reducing the size of the bubbles according to Boyle's law.

Etiology

There are direct (arterial) and indirect (venous) causes of air embolism. Table 9.1 illustrates the etiology of these lesions.

Iatrogenic medical or surgical procedures can introduce gas directly into the arteries. Blunt and penetrating trauma to the thorax also causes gas embolism. Improper catheter flushing or balloon rupture during angioplasty is a risk factor. Injury to the lungs by pressure changes in diving can also lead to embolism. The pressurized venous infusions predispose to venous embolism. Arterial gas embolism occurs during rapid ascent in cases of scuba diving. The cerebral air embolism tends to occur in patients who lack patent foramen ovale.

V. Mago, *Hyperbaric Medicine*, https://doi.org/10.1007/978-981-95-2644-4_9

Table 9.1 Direct and indirect causes of air embolism

Direct entry	Indirect entry
Iatrogenic injury via catheter	Scuba diving
Blast injury	Placement of wrong central venous line
Angioplasty	Hysteroscopic procedures
CABG	Spinal surgery
Lung biopsy	Orogenital sex during pregnancy
Penetrating lung injury	Use of membrane oxygenators
Mechanical ventilation	

Epidemiology

There is an estimated incidence of arterial gas embolism of 1 per 100,000 dives in scuba diving. Deep and long dives are responsible for higher risk. In cardiac surgery, incidence of embolism of 0.003 to 0.007% is seen. The incidence of pulmonary embolism after CABG is 1–4%. Iatrogenic gas embolism has an incidence of 0.03–4%.

Pathoanatomy

There is a route through which air passes in a direct or indirect cause is based on its drag and buoyancy. The volume of air injected can also be lethal. A dose of 200–300 cc of air injected into systemic circulation can lead to death. The volume of bubbles more than 50 cc can obtund the pulmonary circuit leading to an air lock in the ventricles. Larger bubbles obstruct the cerebral circulation leading to ischemia and injury to neurons. Central venous access can lead to debilitating sequelae. Air acts as a foreign body triggering inflammatory reaction and release of chemokines.

Certain factors play an important role in accelerating damage due to arterial gas embolism:

1. Bubble volume—The total volume of air entering the cerebral microvasculature can be 0.12 ml. The time taken for air bubble<38 µm to clear is seconds as compared to a 1 mm bubble which takes 5 hours.
2. Size of bubbles—Cerebral embolism can result with bubbles of size less than 100 µm in size. Weaning after CABG leads to larger bubbles. Large bubbles cause more damage due to rapid obstruction of blood flow.
3. Number of bubbles—more bubbles cause more damage.
4. Blood flow—Increased blood flow in hearts, lungs, and brain tend to incur more damage.

Classification

A. Based on direction of movement of embolus:

1. Orthograde—carried in direction of blood flow.
2. Retrograde—Move opposite from direction of flow due to low specific gravity.
3. Paradoxical—Embolus is carried from venous to arterial side by septal defects or patent foramen ovale.

B. Based on size macro/micro.
C. Based on composition.

1. Thrombotic.
2. Fat droplet.
3. Amniotic fluid.
4. Atherosclerotic.
5. Septic.
6. Air emboli.

D. Based on behaviour -static, dynamic, coalescing.
E. Detection Doppler/echo/CT-MRI Size and location determine the severity of symptoms. Source of entry is critical for prevention and treatment planning.

Clinical Features and Evaluation

The clinical evaluation of a patient based on sudden loss of consciousness or hypovolemic shock should prompt suspicion of venous gas embolism within 10 min of ascent to surface. One should identify the source of air entry, organs involved, and timing of symptom onset.

The assessment is based on the symptoms of respiratory distress (venous air embolism) or neurological (arterial). Patients show altered mental status, headache, dizziness, chest pain, paresthesia, seizures, hemiparesis, aphasia, akinetic mutism, and abnormal Babinski sign.

The diagnostic tests can be a chest X-ray demonstrating air in circulation or signs of pulmonary embolism. Echocardiography detects air in the cardiac chambers and vessels. CT scan reveals air in the brain, right ventricle or pulmonary artery. Figure 9.1 reveals a CT scan of the chest showing pneumomedistinum following chest trauma. Figure 9.2 outlines air embolus in the left occipital lobe.

Effects of HBO

Hyperbaric is useful in cases of AGE as it reduces the size of bubbles both in acute setting and delayed presentations. It is indicated in cases of patients with cardiopulmonary compromise, neurologic defects and end organ damage. It promotes

Fig. 9.1
Pneumomediastinum
following blunt chest
trauma (Green arrow).
Doppler ultrasound is also
helpful to detect gas in the
vasculature

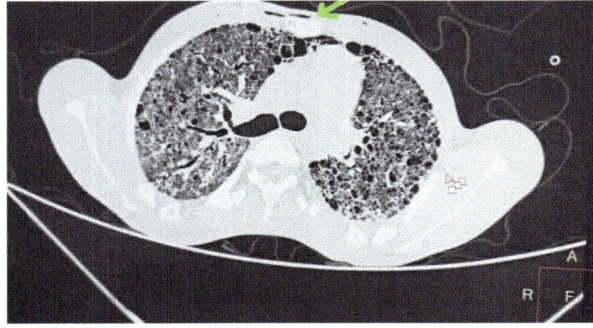

Fig. 9.2 CT scan head
shows air embolus in left
occipital lobe

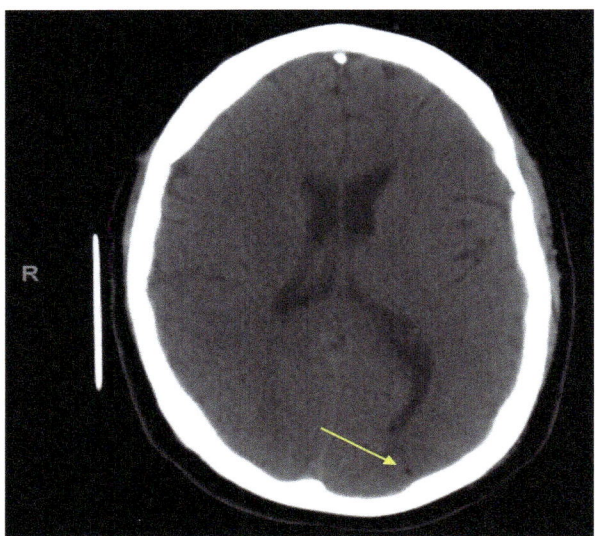

reabsorption of gases based on the gas laws and reduces ischemia perfusion injury. It breaks adhesions between leukocytes and endothelium in affected tissues. As the pressure of the chamber increases, the size of the bubble decreases according to Boyle's law. The principle of Henry's law removes nitrogen by lung excretion once partial pressure of oxygen increases in blood, displacing nitrogen from the bubble. It decreases cerebral edema due to vasoconstriction. It reduces inflammation and ischemia perfusion thus decreasing the deleterious effects of gas embolism on raised icp and brain metabolism.

Dose of HBO

The treatment is initiated as soon as the patient arrives with a pressure of 3 ATA for 30 min, followed by 60 min at 2.4 ATA. The patient returns to baseline after a depth of 120 min. It reduces the size of bubbles, improves blood flow, and reduces the risk of complications. Short monoplace treatment tables should be incorporated in treatment regimens with addition of air breaks. If the symptoms recur, procedure is repeated.

Discussion

Emergency management should be the norm for all physicians to administer 100% oxygen to reduce the size of the bubbles.

Twenty-six patients of arterial air embolism were treated with hyperbaric at a pressure of 280 kPa compression with good outcome in the majority of the patients. Four had minor symptoms which did not affect their quality of life, and 6 developed residual symptoms [1]. The neurological outcomes were good in 27 patients after HBOT, of which 32 patients had arterial source and 13 venous source of emboli [2].

A good favorable outcome in iatrogenic CAGE was found to be 65% in cases with early HBOT vs. 30% if delayed by 15 hours [3]. A patient of cerebral embolism with left sided weakness was given US Navy treatment Table 6 with 100% oxygen at 2.8 ATA for 4 hours 45 min with good functional recovery [4]. Prompt placement in left lateral decubitus position in suspected cases with high flow oxygen is first prerequisite followed by HBOT to improve gas reabsorption [5]. Out of the 16 patients of cerebral air embolism, 8 responded to HBO treatment and 5 received partial relief by mechanical compression of air bubbles to a small size [6].

The physicians should be aware of the role of hyperbaric oxygen therapy in the management of gas embolism. The prevention of iatrogenic incidents can be taught with use of meticulous technique and preserve sanctity of in-dwelling catheters or cvp lines. HBOT prevents reembolisation of brain blood flow, resolve cerebral oedema and decrease bubble size. It facilitates oxygenation of ischemic tissue. HBO is considered a useful modality tp improve tissue oxygenation in compromised blood flow due to bubbles, promote oxygen dissolution by replacing oxygen with nitrogen and expel air emboli from circulation.

References

1. Trytko BE, Bennett MH. Arterial gas embolism: a review of cases at prince of Wales hospital, Sydney, 1996 to 2006. Anaesth Intensive Care. 2008;36(1):60–4.
2. Beevor H, Frawley G. Iatrogenic cerebral gas embolism: analysis of the presentation, management and outcomes of patients referred to the Alfred Hospital hyperbaric unit. Diving Hyperb Med. 2016;46(1):15–21.
3. Fakkert RA, Karlas N, Schober P, Weber NC, Preckel B, van Hulst RA, Weenink RP. Early hyperbaric oxygen therapy is associated with favorable outcome in patients with iatrogenic cerebral arterial gas embolism: systematic review and individual patient data meta-analysis of observational studies. Crit Care. 2023;27(1):282.

4. Murphy RP, Donnellan J. A high-pressure solution for a high-pressure situation: management of Cerebral air Embolism with hyperbaric oxygen therapy. Cureus. 2019;11(9):e5559.
5. Malik N, Claus PL, Illman JE, Kligerman SJ, Moynagh MR, Levin DL, Woodrum DA, Arani A, Arunachalam SP, Araoz PA. Air embolism: diagnosis and management. Futur Cardiol. 2017;13(4):365–78.
6. Murphy BP, Harford FJ, Cramer FS. Cerebral air embolism resulting from invasive medical procedures. Treatment with hyperbaric oxygen. Ann Surg. 1985;201(2):242–5.

Chapter 10
Hyperbaric in Traumatic Brain Injury

Introduction

TBI is a global public health problem affecting 10 million people in the USA. It can be focal or diffuse. Symptomatology varies with area of the brain involved by the injury. Road traffic accidents are a major cause due to lack of using helmets to protect the skull. Lack of access to neurotrauma care in rural areas is the major concern. Lower middle income countries are vulnerable with South East Asia topping the list. HBOT has emerged as a new modality in treatment of TBI due to its neuroprotective effects, reduced apoptosis, protection of blood brain barrier, and anti-inflammatory effects.

Etiology

Main reason is road traffic accidents in low and middle income countries, followed by falls and assaults. Pediatric and elderly patients sustain injuries at home. Rural accidents are more common with a high mortality due to lack of care. Two wheelers account for the majority of the accidents where road safety rules are broken and helmet use is missing.

The causes of TBI are:

1. Falls.
2. Blunt trauma.
3. Vehicle related injuries.
4. Assaults.
5. Explosions or blasts.

V. Mago, *Hyperbaric Medicine*, https://doi.org/10.1007/978-981-95-2644-4_10

Pathophysiology of TBI

Immediate primary injury leads to disruption of neurons, glial cells and blood vessels. After a period of weeks secondary injury sets in with a delayed response of neuronal death characterized by excessive glutamate production and calcium influx. ROS production leads to lipid peroxidation in the brain inciting apoptosis of DNA, lipids and protein. Cerebral oedema and raised ICP occur due to disruption of blood brain barrier. End result is diffuse axonal injury in corpus callosum/brainstem where axonal shearing disrupts communication leading to loss of consciousness. Intracranial haemorrhage increases intracranial pressure.

Classification

Based on Glasgow coma scale:

- Mild.
- Moderate.
- Severe.

Epidemiology

In the USA, 2.5 million suffer from TBI-related emergency visits with 56,000 deaths. India shows an incidence of >1.5 million injuries and 1 million deaths. Maximum injuries are road traffic accidents.

Factors responsible for high incidence are more number of 2-wheelers on the road, lack of road safety, and access to timely care in hospital, especially in rural areas. War veterans also show PTSD, depression, and TBI. Males are more vulnerable to injuries secondary to overzealous driving, alcoholism and work related pressures.

Effects of HBO

The primary effects of TBI are rapid and secondary effects are activated later. HBOT is useful at pressures of 1.5 ATA to exert a neuroprotective effect in mild TBI by giving short and more frequent sessions. It has anti-inflammatory effects by decreasing IL-8 and MMP9. Cerebral edema is reduced by vasoconstriction and proactivates neurons which were damaged by ischemia. The electrical activity in the brain is stimulated by hyperoxygenation. HBOT prevents ammonia toxicity in the brain with glutamine formation and decreases levels of alpha glutarate. Faster rate of compression in diving increases high pressure neurological syndrome. Memory and attention increases in patients given 1.5 ATA hyperbaric therapy. A study conducted by

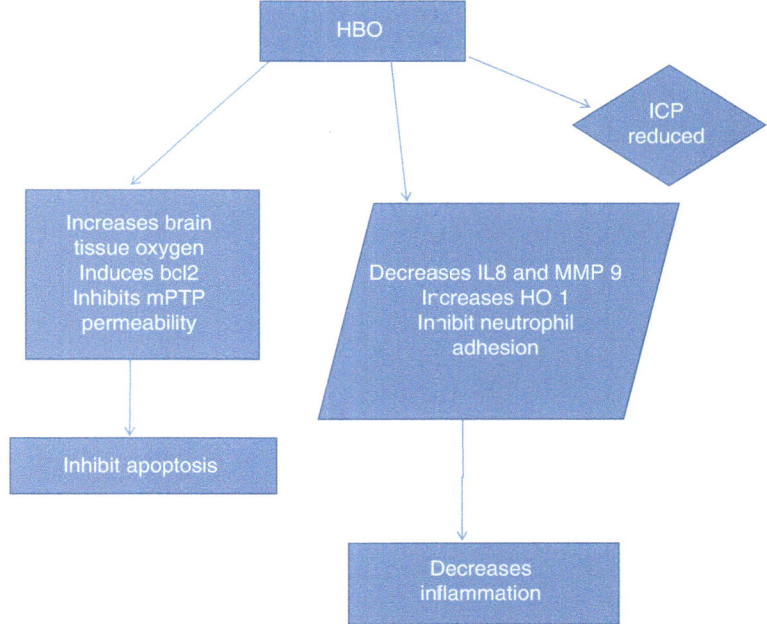

Fig. 10.1 Effects of HBOT

neurosurgery department in our hospital in 10 patients of moderate TBI showed an improvement in GCS score after 10 sessions of 1.4 ATA for 60 min and GOS e scores after 3 months. Growth of new neurons is seen due to reduced apoptosis and increase in mitochondrial function. A flow chart depicts the role of HBOT below (Fig. 10.1)

Discussion

Twelve cases of TBI were treated in this case series with good response seen in patients after diagnosis up to 4 weeks [1]. The results with intensified rehabilitation training with HBO for 2 days improved modified Barthel Index and MMSE scores [2]. Memory domain improved in a cohort of children and improved somatic score and phonemic fluency [3].

HBO led to improvement in sleep quality and balance at 13 weeks after 40 sessions of 1.5 ATA for 60 min [4]. GOS E scores were found to be better at 3 months post injury with HBOT [5]. Patients with GOS 4 improved after 6 months of treatment with HBOT in 22 patients of TBI [6]. GCS scores were found to have increased from 5.1 to 14.6 after 3 sessions and GOS disability rate was 87% [7]. An RCT found 26% reduction in mortality and 36% improvement in GOS scores in 42 patients with severe TBI [8].Veterans with mild TBI and PTSD showed an improvement in SPECT imaging after 40 sessions [9].

Improvement in verbal memory and post-concussive symptoms were seen in patients with TBI who were given HBOT [10]. Angiogenesis is hastened by HBOT, inducing neuroplasticity in post-TBI patients with good global cognitive scores [11]. Functional MRI showed a high brain activity in veterans with PTSD in temporal gyri, bilateral thalami, and insula [12].

The tenets of care in managing cases of TBI are to reduce intracranial pressure and avoid hypotension and hypoxia. Angiogenesis promotes cerebral perfusion in the brain and thus hastens neurogeneration of nerve fibers. It maintains integrity of blood brain barrier. It reactivates dormant neurons improving their function.

References

1. Hajek M, Jor O, Tlapak J, Chmelar D. Hyperbaric oxygen therapy in children with brain injury: a retrospective case series. Int J Med Sci. 2025;22(3):473–81.
2. Lu Y, Zhou X, Cheng J, Ma Q. Early intensified rehabilitation training with hyperbaric oxygen therapy improves functional disorders and prognosis of patients with traumatic brain injury. Adv Wound Care (New Rochelle). 2021;10(12):663–70.
3. Hadanny A, Catalogna M, Yaniv S, Stolar O, Rothstein L, Shabi A, Suzin G, Sasson E, Lang E, Finci S, Polak N, Fishlev G, Harpaz RT, Adler M, Goldman RE, Zemel Y, Bechor Y, Efrati S. Hyperbaric oxygen therapy in children with post-concussion syndrome improves cognitive and behavioral function: a randomized controlled trial. Sci Rep. 2022;12(1):15233.
4. Weaver LK, Wilson SH, Lindblad AS, Churchill S, Deru K, Price RC, Williams CS, Orrison WW, Walker JM, Meehan A, Mirow S. Hyperbaric oxygen for post-concussive symptoms in United States military service members: a randomized clinical trial. Undersea Hyperb Med. 2018;45(2):129–56.
5. Chaturvedi J, Mago V, Gupta M, Singh R, Goyal N, Arora R, Ruchika FNU, Mudgal SK, Gupta P, Agrawal S, Shukla D. Hyperbaric oxygen therapy (HBOT) in moderate traumatic brain injury (TBI): a randomized controlled trial. Asian J Neurosurg. 2024;20(1):69–74.
6. Lin JW, Tsai JT, Lee LM, Lin CM, Hung CC, Hung KS, Chen WY, Wei L, Ko CP, Su YK, Chiu WT. Effect of hyperbaric oxygen on patients with traumatic brain injury. Acta Neurochir Suppl. 2008;101:145–9.
7. Ren H, Wang W, Ge Z. Glasgow coma scale, brain electric activity mapping and Glasgow outcome scale after hyperbaric oxygen treatment of severe brain injury. Chin J Traumatol. 2001;4(4):239–41.
8. Rockswold SB, Rockswold GL, Zaun DA, Liu J. A prospective, randomized phase II clinical trial to evaluate the effect of combined hyperbaric and normobaric hyperoxia on cerebral metabolism, intracranial pressure, oxygen toxicity, and clinical outcome in severe traumatic brain injury. J Neurosurg. 2013;118(6):1317–28.
9. Harch PG, Andrews SR, Fogarty EF, Lucarini J, Van Meter KW. Case control study: hyperbaric oxygen treatment of mild traumatic brain injury persistent post-concussion syndrome and post-traumatic stress disorder. Med Gas Res. 2017;7(3):156–74.
10. Hart BB, Weaver LK, Gupta A, Wilson SH, Vijayarangan A, Deru K, Hebert D. Hyperbaric oxygen for mTBI-associated PCS and PTSD: pooled analysis of results from Department of Defense and other published studies. Undersea Hyperb Med. 2019;46(3):353–83.
11. Tal S, Hadanny A, Berkovitz N, Sasson E, Ben-Jacob E, Efrati S. Hyperbaric oxygen may induce angiogenesis in patients suffering from prolonged post-concussion syndrome due to traumatic brain injury. Restor Neurol Neurosci. 2015;33(6):943–51.
12. Doenyas-Barak K, Catalogna M, Kutz I, Levi G, Hadanny A, Tal S, Daphna-Tekoha S, Sasson E, Shechter Y, Efrati S. Hyperbaric oxygen therapy improves symptoms, brain's microstructure and functionality in veterans with treatment resistant post-traumatic stress disorder: a prospective, randomized, controlled trial. PLoS One. 2022;17(2):e0264161.

Chapter 11
CO Poisoning

Introduction

Carbon monoxide is a byproduct of burning of fuels and is released from automobiles, furnaces, paint strippers, and burning of coal. Expected carboxyhemoglobin levels are 10% in smokers and 5% in nonsmokers. Toxicity is more in cigar smokers. The urban commuters have a level of 5%. It burns with a blue flame. Phosgene gas is produced on combination with chlorine. It is a colorless, odorless and tasteless gas with a specific gravity of 0.6. Coal gas contains 5–7% carbon monoxide. House fires and gas water heaters are a source of CO poisoning in India. Suicidal tendencies in garages is also responsible. The risk factors are enumerated below.

Risk factors of CO poisoning:

- Elderly.
- Infants.
- Pregnancy.
- Emphysema/asthma.
- Anemia/iron deficiency/sickle cell.

Epidemiology

An estimated 50,000 patients report with CO poisoning in the USA. This toxic gas leads to 5000 deaths per year. The rate of non-fire related are >400/year. Forty cases of fatal CO poisoning have been reported in winter months in New Delhi. A crude incidence rate of 1.82 per 100000 people is reported by Global burden of disease(2021). Uttarakhand has reported forest fires leading to CO poisoning and use of fire pots in hilly areas predisposes.

V. Mago, *Hyperbaric Medicine*, https://doi.org/10.1007/978-981-95-2644-4_11

Pathophysiology

On inhalation, it combines with hemoglobin to form carboxyHB which is 200 times more soluble than oxygen. It is a chemical asphyxiant and tissue poison. O2Hb curve shifts to the left which leads to less availability of oxygen in the tissues. CO toxicity is due to cellular hypoxia and tissue toxicity. It affects 3 systems, as shown in Fig. 11.1. CO mostly targets heart and brain.

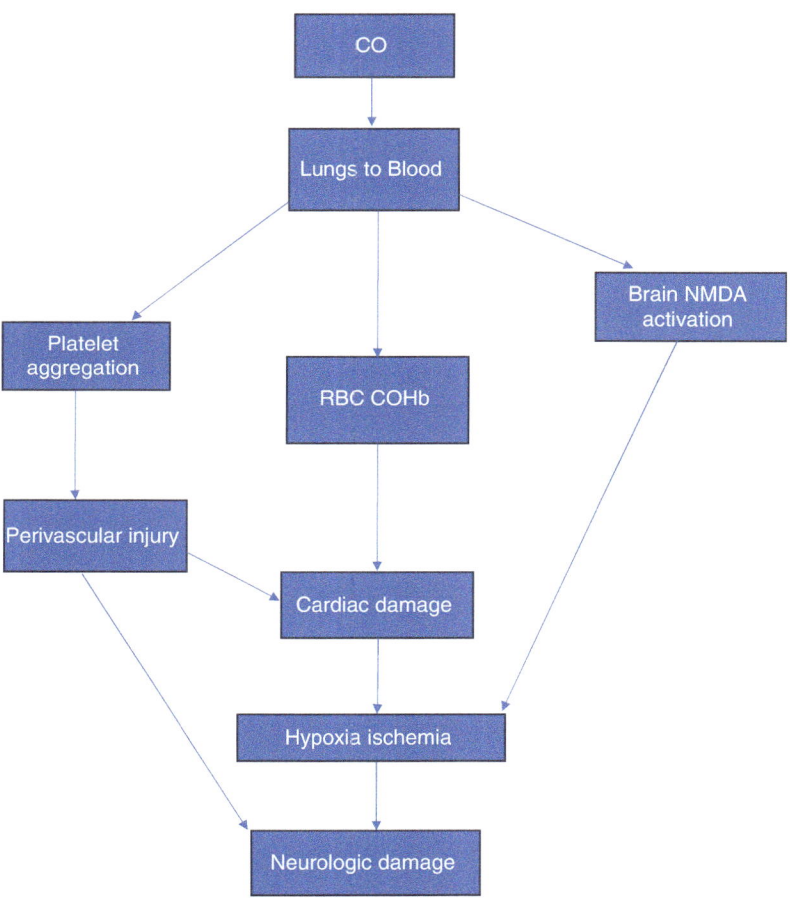

Fig. 11.1 Pathophysiology CO poisoning Effect of CO binding to hemoglobin reduces oxygen transport. Shift of oxygen dissociation curve to left leads to decresed oxygen release in tissues. Mitochondrial binding depletes ATP stores and lipid peroxidation causes cell membrane damage. Anaerobic metabolism is altered by lactic acidosis. CNS and heart become vulnerable to toxicity in form of seizures and coma.

Clinical Features

Two clinical features in acute intoxication are cherry red color of tissues and cutaneous bulla or blisters.

Based on severity:

Mild(COHb<30%).
Moderate(30–40%).
Severe(>40%).
CO levels correlate with the onset of signs and symptoms.
>5% headache
6–10% mild headache with shortness of breath(sOB)
11–20% moderate headache, SOB
21–30% moderate headache, fatigue, nausea, dizziness
31–40% worsening headache, vomiting, vertigo
41–50% confusion, syncope
51–60% seizures, shock, coma, apnea.

Evaluation

Patient is evaluated clinically based on symptoms perceived by severity and COHb levels.

Pulse oximetry and ABG are done. ECG shows depressed ST segments in leads 2, V5 and V6. Chest X-ray measurement of COHb level is by spectrophotometry. CT scan shows areas of low density in globus pallidus.

Effects of HBO

HBOT helps in the removal of carbon monoxide from hemoglobin and cytochrome systems.

Breathing 100% oxygen decreases half-life of CO from 4–6 h to 1–1.5 h. HBO treatment is beneficial in patients with COHb>40%. CO binds to cytochrome oxidase leading to tissue hypoxia. CO binds to myoglobin in muscle causing cardiac damage. HBOT sessions preserve ATP production, increase cytochrome binding, reduce myeloperoxidase activity and induce heat shock proteins. Prevention of brain lipid peroxidation and reduction of necrosis with neuronal apoptosis reverses cognitive decline in patients.

Royal Navy table 60 is used to treat severe CO poisoning with 2 ATA pressure for 90 min with 2 air breaks of 5 min each for 2 hours.

Accelerated elimination of CO prevents lipid peroxidation in brain and preserves ATP in tissue.

Three chambers sessions of 3ATA helps to treat cognitive sequelae. If neurological abnormalities appear, 6 sessions are recommended. The ultimate goal of therapy in CO poisoning is giving 2-3ATA pressure for 60–90 minutes to clear the carbon monoxide. Standard protocol is 3ATA of initial compression, followed by 2ATA for 120 minutes and then 2 sessions of 2ATA for 90 minutes in 6–12 hour intervals. 2–3 treatments are necessary in severe cases for mitigating ischemia perfusion injury. In milder cases only one treatment is lifesaving if given within 6 hours of exposure. Progress is monitored by ECG and measurement of cardiac enzymes Troponin I and creatine kinase MB. Pregnant women and children can be treated with severe poisoning.

Discussion

A total of 102 patients benefitted with HBOT, resulting in mild residual symptoms in 3 patients and mild headache persisted for several weeks [1]. The risk factors noted in this study for mortality issues with CO poisoning were endotracheal intubations, fires, and loss of consciousness [2]. Agitation was seen inside the hyperbaric chamber during the session along with seizures and hypotension. Ten dives were halted to resuscitate patients with 6% mortality rate [3].

Poor outcome is seen in 34 patients with high serum CK levels, low GCS, and long delay in reaching hospital [4].

Neuropsychometric sequelae were less in HBOT treated group [5]. Brain injury in CO poisoning affects cognitive domain, mainly neurological sequelae [6]. Eleven out of 62 patients recovered after DNS with more than 3 HBOT sessions [7]. Accidental causes like gas stove was most common in 12 cases who responded effectively with HBOT with normalization of COHb levels [8]. Nineteen out of 76 patients reported a low level of cognitive effects at 6 weeks with 3 sessions of HBOT [9].

The administration of HBOT brings dramatic improvement in patients with signs of CO poisoning like loss of consciousness, neurological deficit, or recurrent symptoms. It speeds up CO removal and limits delayed brain damage.

References

1. Norkool DM, Kirkpatrick JN. Treatment of acute carbon monoxide poisoning with hyperbaric oxygen: a review of 115 cases. Ann Emerg Med. 1985;14(12):1168–71.
2. Hampson NB, Hauff NM. Risk factors for short-term mortality from carbon monoxide poisoning treated with hyperbaric oxygen. Crit Care Med. 2008;36(9):2523–7.
3. Loan EP, Murphy DG, Hart R, Cooper MA, Turnbull T, Barreca RS, Ellerson B. Complications and protocol considerations in carbon monoxide-poisoned patients who require hyperbaric oxygen therapy: report from a ten-year experience. Ann Emerg Med. 1989;18(6):629–34.

4. Hsu LH, Wang JH. Treatment of carbon monoxide poisoning with hyperbaric oxygen. Zhonghua Yi Xue Za Zhi (Taipei). 1996;58(6):407–13.

5. Lin CH, Su WH, Chen YC, Feng PH, Shen WC, Ong JR, Wu MY, Wong CS. Treatment with normobaric or hyperbaric oxygen and its effect on neuropsychometric dysfunction after carbon monoxide poisoning: a systematic review and meta-analysis of randomized controlled trials. Medicine (Baltimore). 2018;97(39):e12456.

6. Weaver LK. Carbon Monoxide poisoning (reprinted from the 2023 hyperbaric indications manual 15th edition). Undersea Hyperb Med. 2024;51(3):253–76.

7. Liao SC, Shao SC, Yang KJ, Yang CC. Real-world effectiveness of hyperbaric oxygen therapy for delayed neuropsychiatric sequelae after carbon monoxide poisoning. Sci Rep. 2021;11(1):19212.

8. Handa PK, Tai DY. Carbon monoxide poisoning: a five year review at Tan Tock Seng Hospital, Singapore. Ann Acad Med Singap. 2005;34(10):611–4.

9. Weaver LK, Hopkins RO, Chan KJ, Churchill S, Elliott CG, Clemmer TP, Orme JF Jr, Thomas FO, Morris AH. Hyperbaric oxygen for acute carbon monoxide poisoning. N Engl J Med. 2002;347(14):1057–67.

Chapter 12
Compromised Flaps and Grafts

Introduction

Grafts and flaps are tissues transferred from one part of the body to another for reconstructing lost body parts or surfaces. A flap is a piece of tissue with intact blood supply. A graft is a piece of tissue which is detached from site of origin and transferred to a different site. A graft can be any tissue comprising fascia, muscle nerve, vessel, bone, cartilage, and composite tissue. Mastectomy skin flap necrosis is a complication of mastectomy in 2–30% cases worldwide.

It takes approximately three days for capillaries to develop in a newly placed graft over a wound bed. If the graft or flap becomes hypoxic during this time, risk for flap failure increases markedly.

Factors leading to compromised flaps are:

1. Impaired perfusion of the flap.
   In irradiated tissues and burns, survival of a flap is improved by hyperbaric therapy in providing neovascularization. Burns lead to extracellular fluid losses compromising graft healing. Increased oxygen carrying capacity of the plasma prevents ongoing tissue necrosis. Gaped abdominal wounds heal faster exemplifying their role (Figs. 12.1 and 12.2).
2. Infections.
   Burn patients are exposed to a myriad of infections as skin barrier is lost and immune status is compromised. HBOT lowers the bacterial burden by its bateriostatic properties and bactericidal effects on microorganisms. An increase in the oxygen tension kills exotoxins (Figs. 12.3 and 12.4).

V. Mago, *Hyperbaric Medicine*, https://doi.org/10.1007/978-981-95-2644-4_12

Fig. 12.1 Gaped
abdominal wound

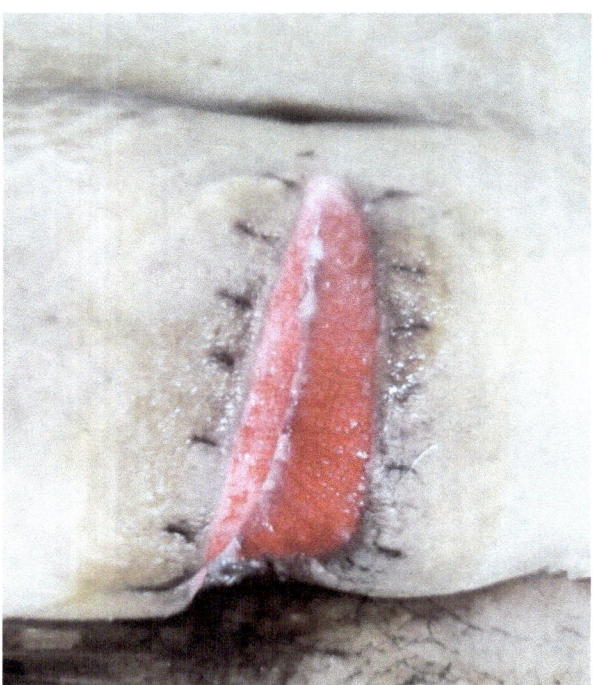

Fig. 12.2 Healed
abdominal wound
after HBOT

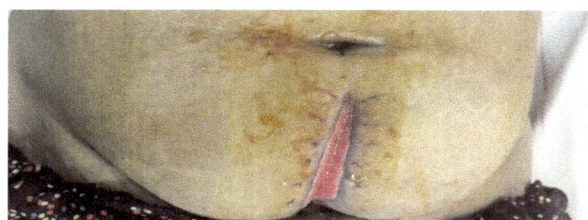

3. Vascular compromise.

   Delayed flap healing is due to poor vascularity, surgical techniques, and patient factors (Figs. 12.5 and 12.6). The risk factors for delayed graft uptake at donor sites of free ALT flap are high BMI, smoking, and tobacco chewing.

4. Delayed intervention—It refers to improving flap survival under unfavorable conditions.

Fig. 12.3 Infected thermal burns over right leg

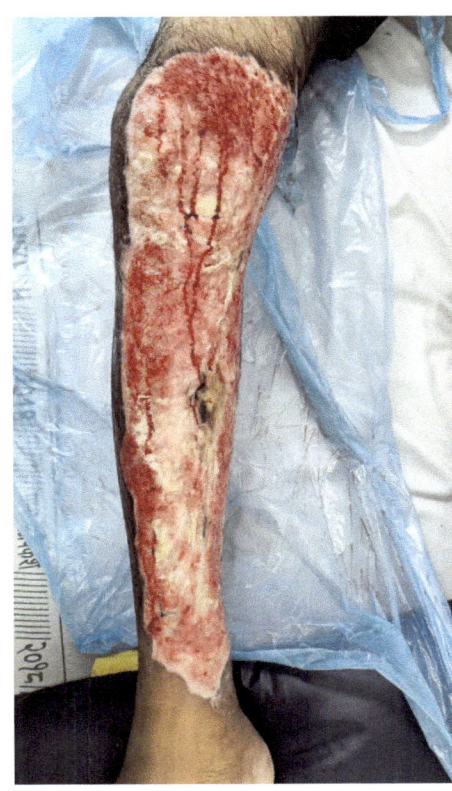

Fig. 12.4 After 10 HBOT cycles, infection curbed and wound bed prepared

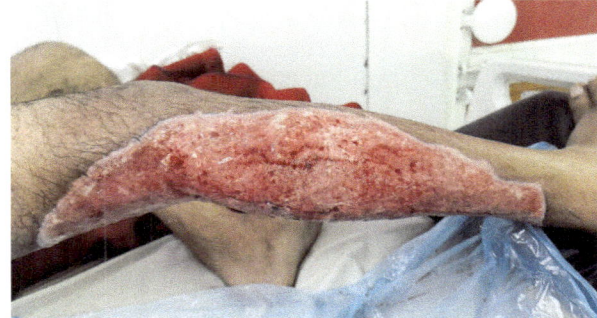

Fig. 12.5 Compromised
pedicled radial forearm
flap of right hand

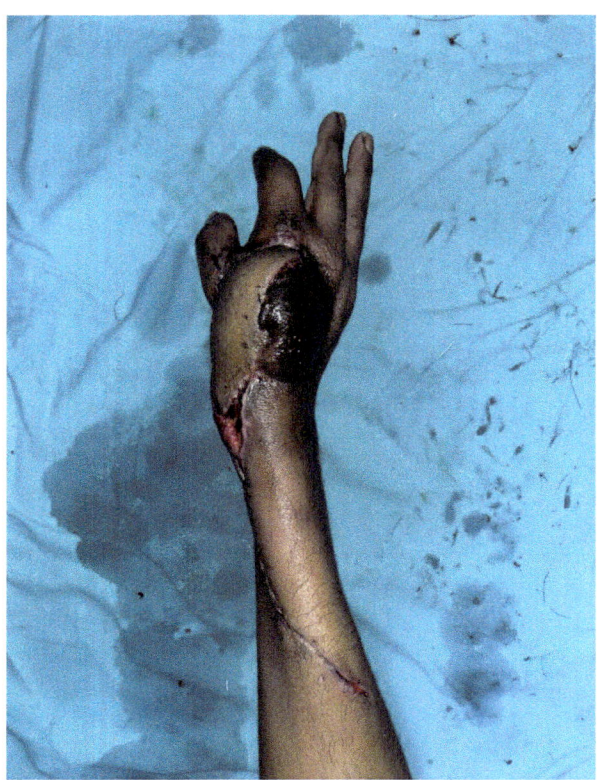

Fig. 12.6 Flap survived
after 10 cycles of HBOT

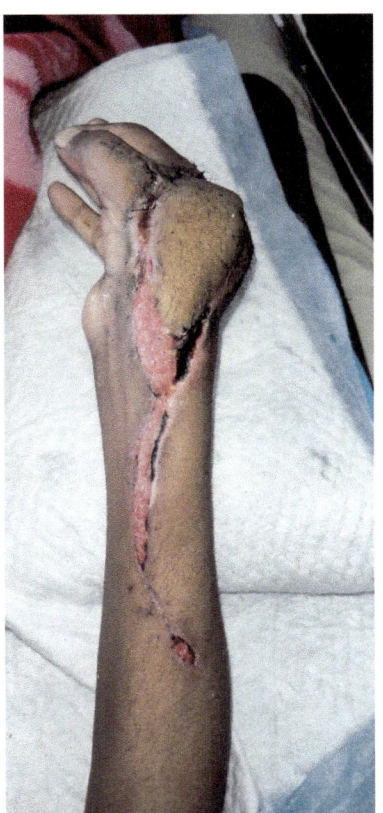

Classification

Skin Grafts

Skin grafts are transplanted from one area of the body to another. Skin grafts can be split thickness or full thickness. It helps to restore skin integrity.

A. According to skin thickness:

   1. Split thickness.

      Thin (0.2–0.3 mm).
      Intermediate (0.3–0.45 mm).
      Thick(0.45–0.6 mm) (Fig. 12.7).

   2. Full thickness.
      Fully detached pieces of skin are transferred from one site to another. It includes full epidermis and dermis (Fig. 12.8).

Fig. 12.7 Split thickness skin grafting for medial malleolar ulcer

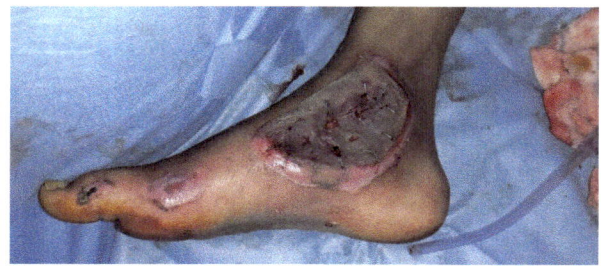

Fig. 12.8 Full thickness grafts placed on contracture release over left hand

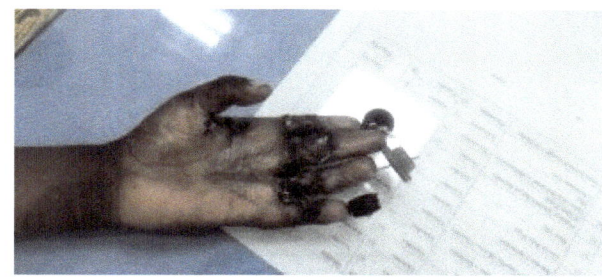

B. According to their origin:

   Autografts—same individual.
   Homografts—different individual.
   Xenografts—different species.

C. Based on type or pattern sheet:

   Island—postage stamp or punch or strip.
   Based on meshing—Meshed (Fig. 12.6) or unmeshed.

Flaps

Based on 7 Cs they are classified as

1. Components.

   Cutaneous—it comprises skin and superficial fascia.
   Fascial—includes deep fascia.
   Fasciocutaneous—skin and deep fascia.
   Muscle—Gastrocnemius muscle flap is used to cover upper third leg defects (Fig. 12.9).
   Bone—fibula, scapula, iliac crest.
   Visceral—sigmoid, jejunum.
   Innervated—functional or sensory flaps.
   Complex (Fig. 12.9).

Fig. 12.9 Gastrocnemius
muscle flap with skin graft

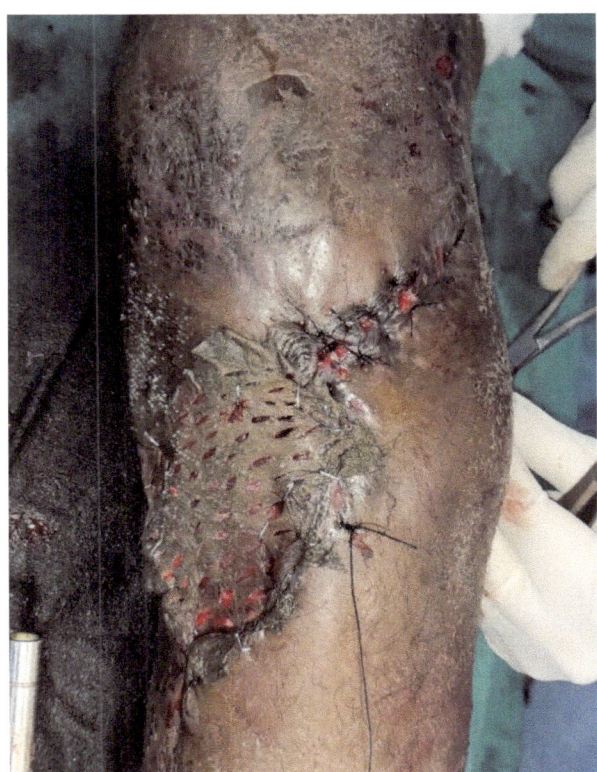

Fig. 12.10 Bilobed flap
over nose (random)

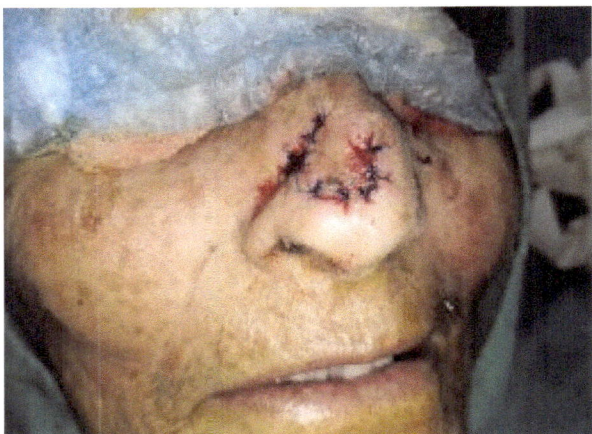

2. Circulation.

   Random—These flaps rely on subdermal vascular plexus. Examples are the
   rhomboid flap and bilobed flaps (Fig. 12.10).

Axial—A flap based on a named arterial supply. Forehead axial flap is based on the supratrochlear artery (Fig. 12.7). Radial artery forearm flap is an axial flap based on the radial artery (Fig. 12.6).

3. Method of moving—Configuration.

Advancement—These flaps are sliding flaps where tissue is moved into adjacent defect (Fig. 12.11).

Rotation—These flaps rotate around a pivot point to close a primary defect (Fig. 12.14a, b).

Transposition—They switch positions of 2 or more areas of tissue to close defects like Z plasties (Fig. 12.12).

Fig. 12.11 Mustarde advancement flap

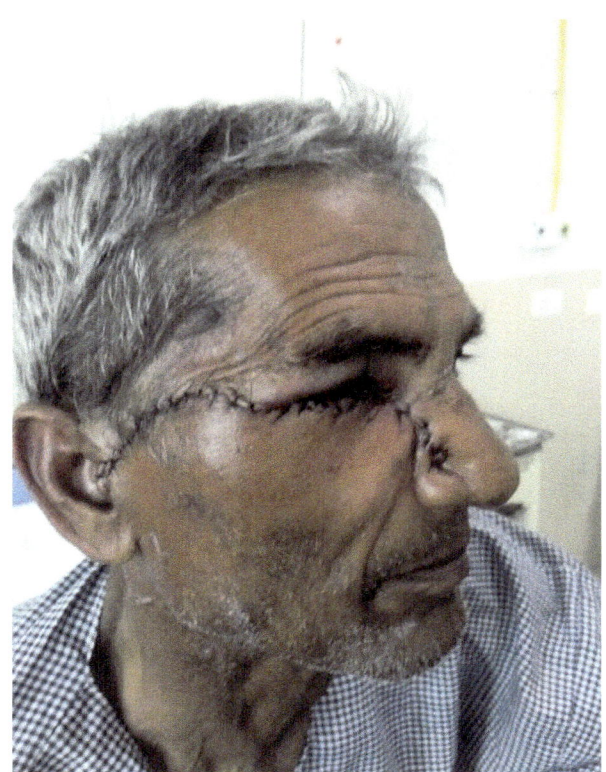

Fig. 12.12 Transposition fasciocutaneous flap upper one third leg defect

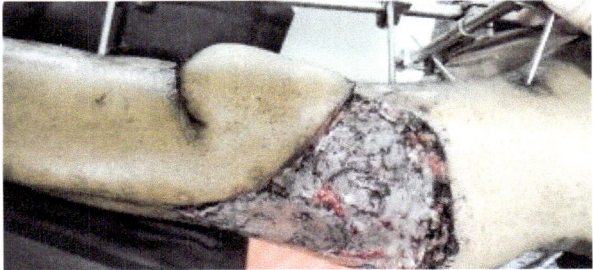

Fig. 12.13 Forehead interpolation flap

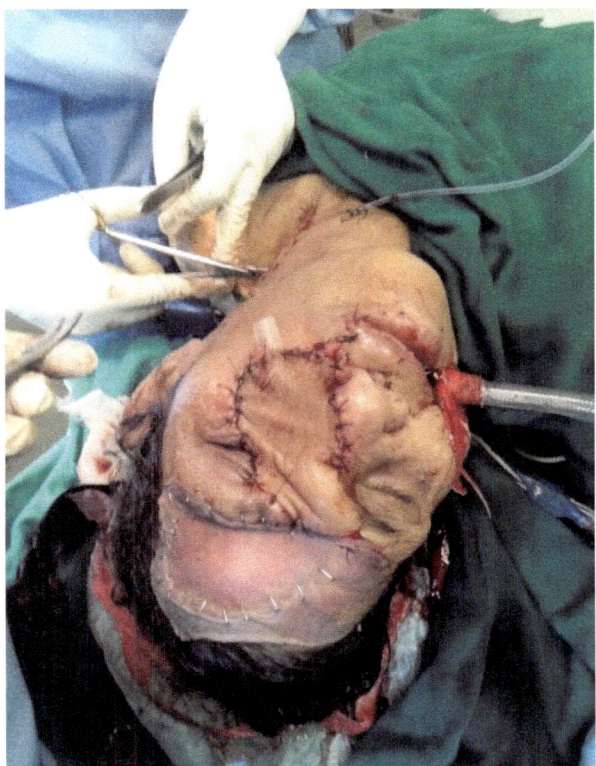

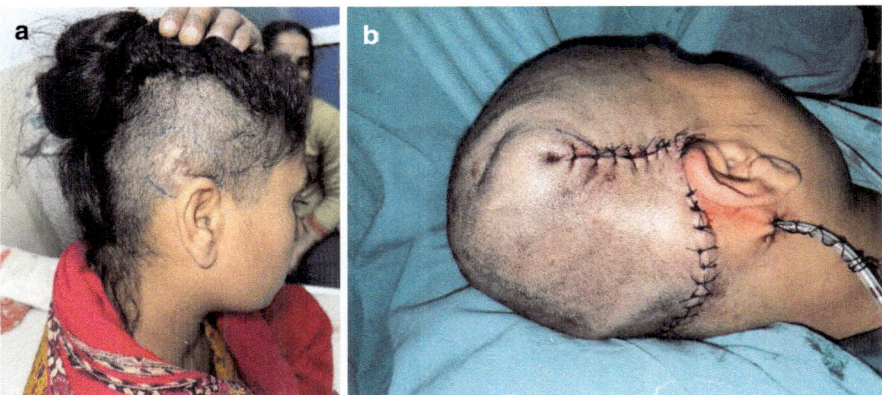

Fig. 12.14 (**a**) Squamous cell carcinoma temporal region scalp. (**b**) Rotation scalp flap into defect

Interpolation—This is a flap whose pedicle traverses over a segment of normal tissue (Fig. 12.13). The base is located away from the defect (Fig. 12.14).

Island—It involves transposition of an island of skin based on its blood supply. It is useful to cover defects over nose, ears, and periorbital areas.

Hinged—These flaps turn over like pages of a book to cover defects. Septal hinge flap is useful to cover defects over ala, tip, and sidewalls.

4. Composition.

Skin.
Superficial fascia.
Deep fascia.
Muscle.
Bone.

5. Construction.

Retrograde—It relies on retrograde flow through artery of the pedicle like sural flap (Fig. 12.15). Retrograde posterior interosseous flap is another option for hand defects.

Turbocharged—This flap allows more blood flow to remote areas of the flap. Renal transplantation involves turbocharging by anastomosing accessory renal artery to main renal artery with a vascular graft.

Venous—These flaps are useful in the repair of defects with segmental vessel loss. The saphenous venous flap is an example of this flap.

Unipedicled or bipedicled—This flap is seen in TRAM flap for breast reconstruction based on one pedicle or bipedicle.

Fig. 12.15 Retrograde flow sural flap

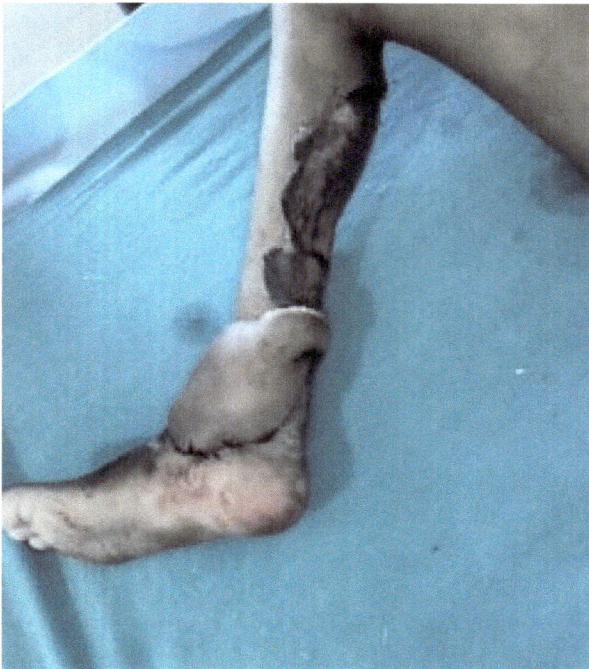

Fig. 12.16 Free DIEP flap over right breast

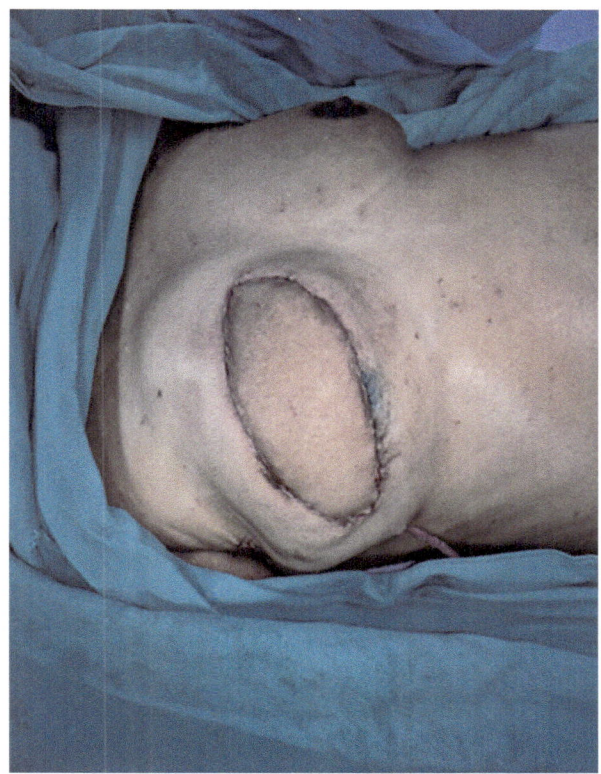

6. Conditioning.

   Delay—It is the method of increasing vascular territory of a flap by surgical or chemical ways (Fig. 12.16).

   Tissue expansion—A tissue expander increases additional skin and soft tissue to reconstruct defects. The areas like the scalp can be reinforced with expanders to cover defects over scalp (Fig. 12.17).

7. Contiguity.

   Local-flap lies next to defect.

   Regional-flap in same region as defect.

   Distant-flap is far away from defect.

   Free-Various types of tissues can be transferred as free flaps. Free DIEP flap is a viable option for breast reconstruction after mastectomy (Fig. 12.16).

Fig. 12.17 Showing tissue
expander in place over the
scalp

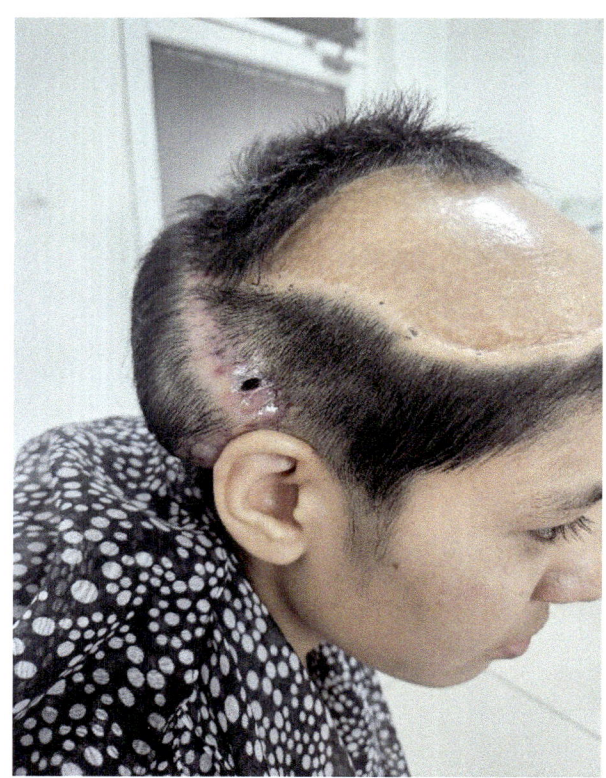

Benefits of Hyperbaric

The compromised flaps are undergoing both ischemic and reperfusion injury, which
can also be attenuated by HBOT to maximize viability.

It increases oxygen supply over the entire free or pedicled flap. When wound
edges are devascularised, HBO enhances wound closure (Fig. 12.3).

Hyperbaric oxygen therapy has been found to be useful in our center for possible
intervention for threatened flaps in operative procedures.

Even free flaps can be salvaged with hyperbaric therapy. Tissue edema in free
flaps is reduced after 5 sessions. Free flaps are prone to IR injury, arterial insufficiency, or venous thrombosis.

HBOT possessed a bactericidal effect on anaerobic infection.

HBO increased superoxide anion production by macrophages and likely kills
bacteria by oxidative mechanisms.

Fig. 12.18 Raw area right forearm with external fixator

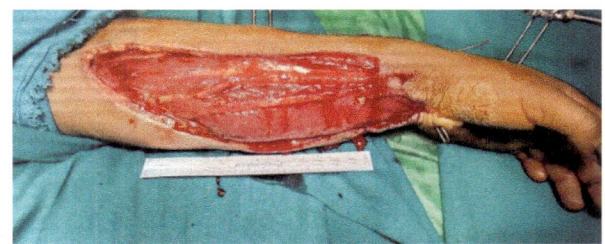

Fig. 12.19 POD with 95–100% uptake of skin graft after second HBOT cycle

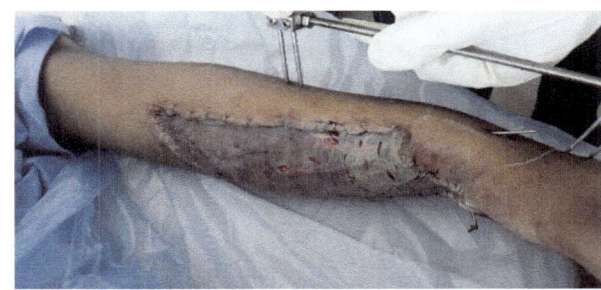

It mitigates the effects of ischemia perfusion injury.

HBOT cause the potentiation of antibiotics by enhancing its uptake and effectiveness.

HBOT improves collagen production in areas of wound hypoxia.

A thesis was done on utility of HBOT on the salvage of skin grafts in trauma patients which revealed excellent results on graft uptake after fifth HBOT session and subsequent 15th session of HBOT. The chances of regrafting were minimal after HBOT.

The probability of survival of skin grafts is accelerated by HBOT through increased production of collagen by the fibroblasts. There is an increase in number of capillaries which accounts for the bridging phenomenon seen in full thickness grafts who survive in avascular beds. Secondary revascularization sets in once ischemic period is extended beyond tolerance of graft (Figs. 12.18 and 12.19).

Compromised flaps are salvaged if HBOT is instituted early and favors delivery of oxygen from plasma which restores tissue hypoxia and increases perfusion by stimulating angiogenesis (Fig. 12.20a, b). Venous congestion is the most common cause for failure of free flaps. Pedicle flaps can fail due to mechanical occlusion. HBOT helps by delivery of oxygen through perforators present in musculocutaneous or septocutaneous plane in compromised pedicle flaps where mechanical occlusion has been excluded(Figs. 12.21 and 12.22). The vascular supply of random flaps improves by primary revascularization by hyperbaric oxygen therapy.

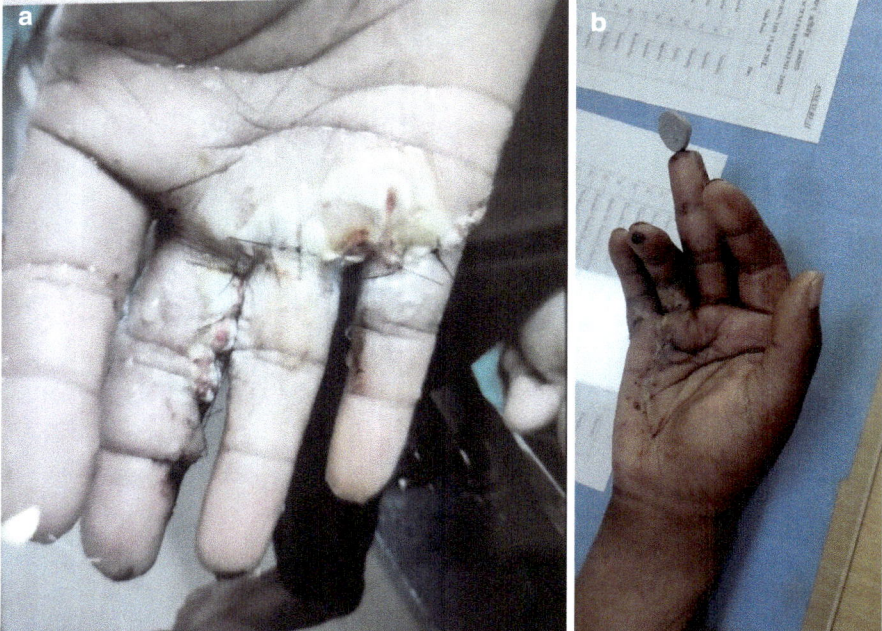

Fig. 12.20 (**a**) Post-trauma compromised flaps right hand. (**b**) Healed tissues right hand after 10 cycles of HBOT

Fig. 12.21 Compromised proximal based sural flap over right knee (yellow arrow head)

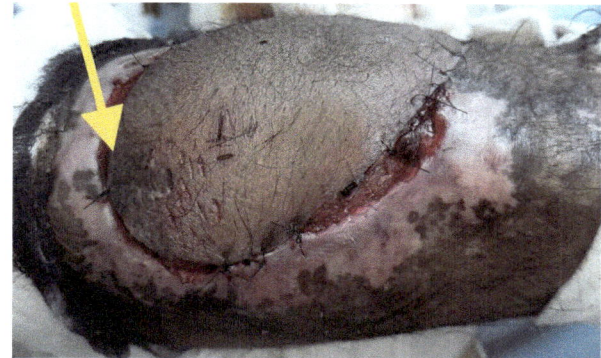

Dose of HBO

Ten HBOT sessions are administered over the course of 2 weeks at 2.4 atmospheres (2.4 bar O2 /90 min) for compromised flaps. Therapeutic effect depends on the progress of resolving compromise, reduction of tissue oedema or graft uptake. The skin graft uptake improves after 2–5 sessions.

Fig. 12.22 Flap salvage after HBOT

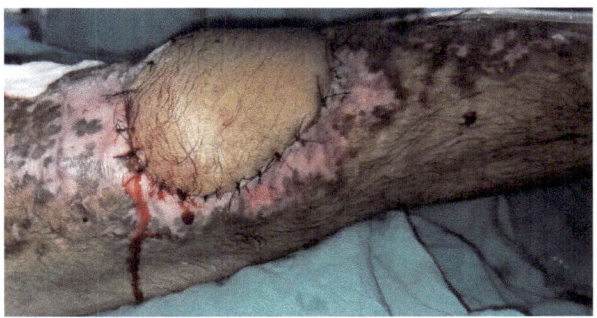

Discussion

Neovascularization is a prerequisite for donor tissue to survive.

HBO treatment was associated with vimentin immunoreactivity in fibroblasts, endothelial cells, and the bulbous pilorum of a subset of hair follicles. It also resulted in increased type IV collagen expression in rat facial skin [1].

Skin grafts are at a high risk of lipid peroxidation on exposure to hyperbaric [2].

Animal studies have demonstrated an increase in blood supply by hyperbaric oxygen therapy [3].

The expedient initiation of hyperbaric oxygen therapy as soon as flap or graft compromise is identified maximizes tissue viability and ultimately graft/flap salvage [4].

The utilization of leech therapy (*Hirudo medicinalis*) with HBO2 in a compromised breast flap promises a better outcome than each modality alone [5].

All patients manifested successful healing of their mastectomy skin flaps with acceptable cosmesis after 10 HBO2 treatments [6]. ICGA is a useful adjunct for evaluating post-mastectomy breast flap perfusion before and after HBO2 therapy.

Hyperbaric oxygen therapy indications included ischemia or venous congestion for 15 breasts (60.0%) and partial thickness necrosis for 10 breasts (40.0%). Flap salvage was achieved in 22 of 25 breasts (88.0%). Reoperation was required for 3 breasts [7].

HBOT is efficacious for mitigating post-NMS complications, including infections, re-operation, flap loss, seroma, and hematoma [8].Within this early-intervention subgroup of breast nipple sparing mastectomy, a 90% success rate was seen in 10 cases of resolving threatened skin flap necrosis patients. 8 patients had improvement in healing of breast NAC complex with a faster healing in HBOT group [9].

HBOT achieved wound vascular regeneration in healing keratinized oral mucosal flaps, resulting from a significant increase in microcirculation in the HBOT group relative to the control group on days 7, 9, and 11 [10]. Skin rejuvenation with improvement in wrinkles is seen with hyperbaric therapy by stimulating angiogenesis through HIF 1 alpha, VEGF and MMP 9 pathways [11].

HBO in combination with imipenem can be used to kill *P. aeruginosa* in vitro and potentiate role of imipenem in combating infections [12].

The ptcO2 values increased significantly from 42.59 ± 1.11 Torr before to 81.14 ± 5.95 Torr after hyperbaric treatment ($p < 0.001$). Even after 2 hours the ptcO2 values were significantly higher in free flaps treated by hyperbaric [13].

In this study, all avulsed ears were reattached along with three nose avulsions and composite ear grafts were used. HBO was initiated immediately and continued for 8–10 days. All grafts survived, at least 80% with no postoperative complications [14].

Seven boys of hypospadias cripples received HBOT and 14 boys comprised the control group. All patients in the HBOT group had good graft take with no graft contraction [15]. This study emphasized that 20 sessions can induce angiogenesis in hypospadias cripples.

Increased VEGF levels are seen in rats receiving HBO therapy for 7 days which is responsible for angiogenesis [16]. HBO treatment increased the percentage of survival length and mean LD flows of axial pattern skin flaps with all types of vascular insufficiency. This effect, however, was greatest in the arterial insufficiency flaps [17]. Hyperbaric therapy has reversed impending flap necrosis in 2 patients and hastened survival of full thickness grafts once skin grafts fail [18]. Patients in this study underwent wide and deep periorbital excisions with eight adjunctive sessions of HBO therapy in patients with basal cell carcinoma. Five cases of post surgery wound healing in basal cell carcinoma cases treated by transposition flap improved with 8 sessions of HBO [19]. This is the first published case of survival of SGAP-free flap for right breast reconstruction after 17 sessions of HBOT [20].

HBOT is useful to salvage compromised tissue once the subacute process of ischemic necrosis has begun. Hyperbaric oxygen decreases local tissue edema and improves oxygen delivery to compromised tissues. Hyperbaric oxygen therapy reduces the need for regrafting. It improves survival of free flaps. HBOT reduces financial, physical and mental costs of failing pedicled or free flaps and reduces need for secondary surgeries.

References

1. Sula B, Ekinci C, Uçak H, et al. Effects of hyperbaric oxygen therapy on rat facial skin. Hum Exp Toxicol. 2015;35(1):35–40.
2. Lemarié RJ, Hosgood G, VanSteenhouse J, et al. Effect of hyperbaric oxygen on lipid peroxidation in free skin grafts in rats. Am J Vet Res. 1998;59:913–7.
3. Gould LJ, May T. The science of hyperbaric oxygen for flaps and grafts. Surg Technol Int. 2016;28:65–72.
4. Baynosa RC, Zamboni WA. The effect of hyperbaric oxygen on compromised grafts and flaps. Undersea Hyperb Med. 2012;39(4):857–65.

5. Moffat AD, Weaver LK, Tettelbach WH. Compromised breast flap treated with leech therapy, hyperbaric oxygen, pentoxifylline and topical nitroglycerin: a case report. Undersea Hyperb Med. 2015;42(3):281–4.

6. Rajpal N, Walters ET, Elmarsafi T, Pittman TA, Johnson-Arbor KK. Use of hyperbaric oxygen therapy for tissue ischemia after breast reconstruction. Undersea Hyperb Med. 2019;46(4):461–5.

7. Nasr HY, Rifkin WJ, Muller JN, Chiu ES. Hyperbaric oxygen therapy for threatened nipple-sparing mastectomy flaps: an adjunct for flap salvage. Ann Plast Surg. 2023;90(5S Suppl 2):S125–9.

8. Idris OA, Ahmedfiqi YO, Shebrain A, Al-Assil T, Pacione SC, Haj D, Motan AD, Momani F, Bzizi H, Jahromi BS, Lewis RM, Steeg KV 2nd. Hyperbaric oxygen therapy for complications in nipple-sparing mastectomy with breast reconstruction: a systematic review. J Clin Med. 2024;13(12):3535.

9. Shuck J, O'Kelly N, Endara M, Nahabedian MY. A critical look at the effect of hyperbaric oxygen on the ischemic nipple following nipple-sparing mastectomy and implant-based reconstruction: a case series. Gland Surg. 2017;6:659–65.

10. Helmers R, Milstein DM, van Hulst RA, et al. Hyperbaric oxygen therapy accelerates vascularization in keratinized oral mucosal surgical flaps. Head Neck. 2014;36:1241–7.

11. Asadamongkol B, Zhang JH. The development of hyperbaric oxygen therapy for skin rejuvenation and treatment of photoaging. Med Gas Res. 2014;4(1):7.

12. Lima FL, Joazeiro PP, Lancellotti M, de Hollanda LM, de Araújo LB, Linares E, Augusto O, Brocchi M, Giorgio S. Effects of hyperbaric oxygen on Pseudomonas aeruginosa susceptibility to imipenem and macrophages. Future Microbiol. 2015;10(2):179–89.

13. Gehmert S, Geis S, Lamby P, et al. Evaluation of hyperbaric oxygen therapy for free flaps using planar optical oxygen sensors. Preliminary results. Clin Hemorheol Microcirc. 2011;48(1–3):75–9.

14. Camison L, Naran S, Lee WW, Grunwaldt LJ, Davit AJ, Goldstein JA, O'Toole KS, Losee JE, Adetayo OA. Hyperbaric oxygen therapy for large composite grafts: an alternative in pediatric facial reconstruction. J Plast Reconstr Aesthet Surg. 2020;73(12):2178–84.

15. Neheman A, Rappaport YH, Verhovsky G, Bush N, Snodgrass W, Lang E, Zisman A, Efrati S. Hyperbaric oxygen therapy for pediatric "hypospadias cripple"-evaluating the advantages regarding graft take. J Pediatr Urol. 2020;16(2):163.e1–7.

16. Sheikh AY, Gibson JJ, Rollins MD, Hopf HW, Hussain Z, Hunt TK. Effect of hyperoxia on vascular endothelial growth factor levels in a wound model. Arch Surg. 2000;135:1293–7.

17. Ulkur E, Yuksel F, Acikel C, Celikoz B. Effect of hyperbaric oxygen on pedicle flaps with compromised circulation. Microsurgery. 2002;22:16–20.

18. Gonnering RS, Kindwall EP. Goldmann adjunct hyperbaric oxygen therapy in periorbital reconstruction. Arch Ophtalmol. 1986;104(3):439–43.

19. Oley MH, Oley MC, Gunawan DF, Rangan AA, Wagiu AMJ, Faruk M. Adjunctive hyperbaric oxygen therapy with reconstruction of lower eyelid for basal cell carcinoma: a case series. Int J Surg Case Rep. 2023;103:107890.

20. Park SK, Schank KJ, Engwall-Gill A, Clarkson JHW. Superior gluteal artery perforator flap salvaged via hyperbaric oxygen therapy. BMJ Case Rep. 2022;15(3):e248411.

Chapter 13
Hyperbaric in Necrotizing Fasciitis

Introduction

NSTI or flesh-eating disease encompasses a series of diseases including necrotizing fasciitis, necrotizing cellulitis, Fournier's gangrene, and gas gangrene, in which the conditions may have different microbiological etiologies or anatomical sites. The annual incidence of NSTI varies considerably but is often reported at approximately four per 100,000 in developed countries. It has a mortality rate of 20–40%.

The most common sites involved are the perineum and extremities. Patients residing in the southern part of America had the worst outcomes, being uninsured and with more incidence of clostridial infections.

Staphylococcus aureus was the most common organism globally, followed by streptococcus and E. Coli.

The initial event in the onset of NSTI is the introduction of bacteria into the soft tissues through trauma (accidental or surgical) or spontaneously without a defined portal of entry. NSTI, if not treated, can be rapidly fatal. Cellulitis most commonly occurs in lower limbs (Fig. 13.3). It can be secondary to subjacent infections like abscesses, fistulas, or osteomyelitis.

Fournier's gangrene involves the genital, anal, or perianal regions with a high mortality rate. *E coli* and *pseudomonas* are the most common organisms in wound cultures. This disease is more common in males (Fig. 13.1). Pathophysiology of this disease is bacterial translocation, leading to formation of enzymes, collagenases, and toxins that leads to massive tissue destruction. The classic finding of Fournier's is severe pain out of proportion to the physical findings. Early and radical surgery, broad spectrum antibiotics, and intensive care support remain the cornerstone of treatment.

V. Mago, *Hyperbaric Medicine*, https://doi.org/10.1007/978-981-95-2644-4_13

Fig. 13.1 Fournier's
gangrene of right and left
testes and extending up to
right thigh

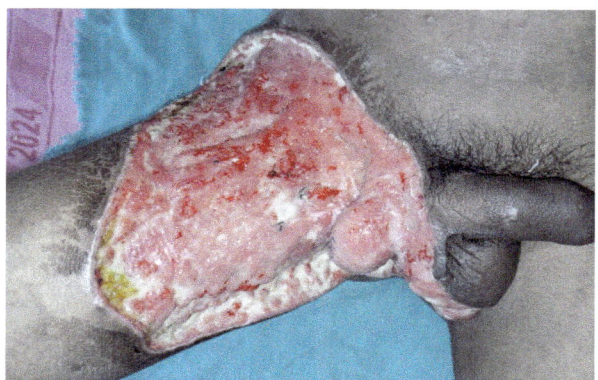

Pathophysiology

The vicious cycle of infection,toxin production,ischemia and host response leads to tissue necrosis and systemic sepsis.Upper limbs harbour group A streptococci and Staph aureus at portal of entry whereas lower limbs have clostridia and group C streptococci.Generation of exotxins leads to thrombi formation in peripheral arteries leading to hypoperfusion,ischemia and necrosis.

Risk Factors

Diabetes is a very common precipitating cause of this fulminating disease (Fig. 13.2). Increased prevalence of obesity is another risk factor. Chronic immunosuppression or intake of steroids is another notable risk factor. Other risk factors are burns, alcoholism, smoking, drug use, and hypothyroidism seen in cervicofacial region. Risk factors like immunosuppression, upper extremity infection, and elevated serum sodium concentration were associated with monomicrobial infection, whereas morbid obesity and perineal infections were associated with polymicrobial infection (Fig. 13.3).

Fig. 13.2 Post diabetes necrotizing cellulitis right foot with amputated fourth toe

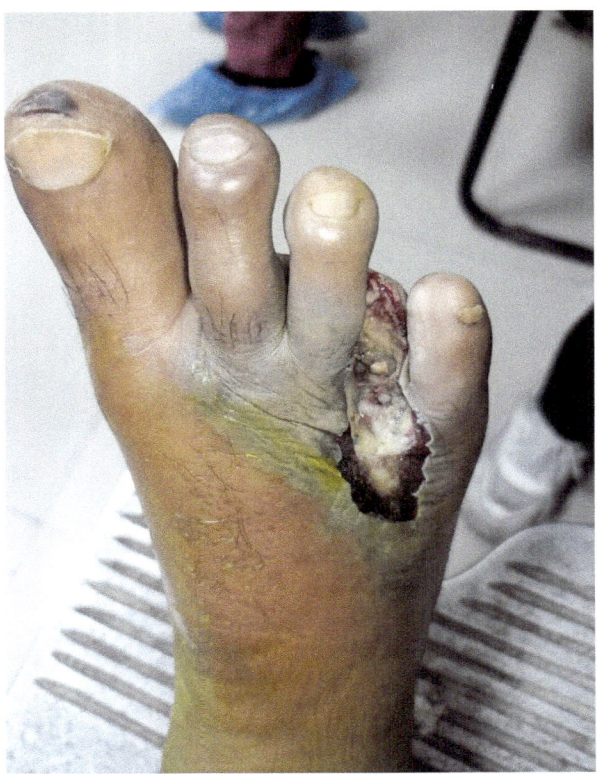

Fig. 13.3 Post venous
ulcer cellulitis right leg
with hyperpigmentation

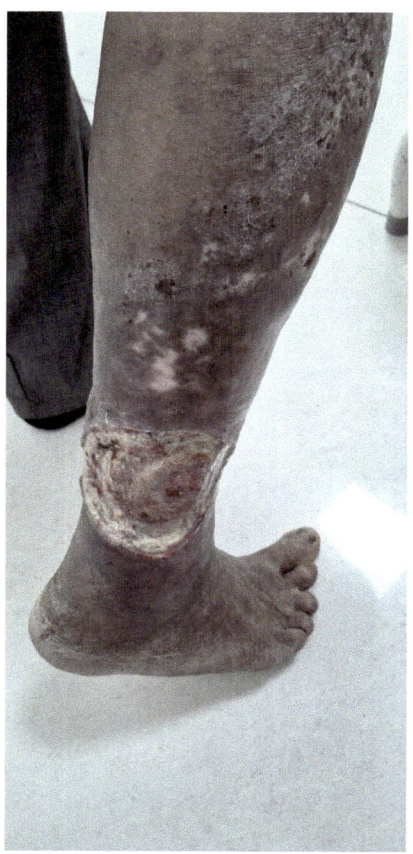

Physiologic Basis of HBO

When oxygen is administered at >1 ATA it becomes a drug and exerts a beneficial effect on cellular metabolism, tissue repair, and promotes host defenses. It also leads to increased tissue oxygen tension. This superoxygenated zone creates an aura to cure fulminating infections and promote healing. There is damping of the systemic inflammatory response. It preserves tissue and decreases the number of debridements. With the increase in tissue PO_2 formed with the effect of H_2O_2, superoxide anions, and oxygen radicals, a bactericidal and bacteriostatic effect is created. The phagocytosis by polymorphs and macrophages is increased. Toxic production of bacteria is halted. By increasing the mucopolysaccharide structure, angiogenesis is accelerated. Tissue edema decreases. Collagen production and fibroblastic activity increases and enhances immunity.

Table 13.1 Infectious causes related indications of HBOT

Infectious causes	Non-infective causes
Gas gangrene	Air embolism
Intracranial abscess	CO poisoning
Necrotizing soft tissue infections	Decompression sickness
Refractory osteomyelitis	Idiopathic sensorineural deafness
	Arterial insufficiency

Indications for HBOT in Infective Causes

HBOT has proved a boon for treating infections like gas gangrene, intracranial abscess, and necrotizing fasciitis. Based on the plethora of mechanisms of its beneficial roles in various indications, Table 13.1 illustrates the various infective indications approved for treatment in a hyperbaric chamber.

Patient Selection and Evaluation

The indications of hyperbaric are confirmed cases with extensive infection, involvement of perineum and cervicofacial and diabetic patients. All patients with NSTI should be evaluated for underlying upper respiratory or cardiopulmonary disease, and seizures may be precipitated depending upon the patient's history. Any history of brain, ear, or thoracic surgery should be ruled out. Hemodynamically unstable patients should not be treated with HBO. Multiplace chambers allow closer monitoring of critically ill patients, whereas monoplace chambers are most appropriate for the treatment of chronic medical conditions in stable patients. Surgical debridement is the mainstay of NSTI treatment. All affected tissue should be sharply excised with at least 1 cm rim of normal tissue. The large soft tissue defects that result from appropriate debridement of NSTI will require extensive reconstructive procedures or skin grafting once the patient has recovered from the acute episode. Table 13.2 shows the number of published articles which have benefitted with HBOT therapy till date. Clinical evaluation is done by hemogram, CRP and renal profile. Ultrasound/CT/MRI reveals fluid thickening and gas. Cultures from deep tissue clinch the diagnosis.

Table 13.2 Published journal articles of NSTI and HBO

Author	Year	Design	HBO	Control	Outcome
Devaney et al.	2015	Retrospective	275	66	Improved outcome
Thrane et al. [9]	2017	Retrospective	30	13	Optional treatment
Flanagan et al. [10]	2009	Case series	10	–	Decreased hospital stay
Kornohen [5]	1998	Retrospective	33	–	Reduced systemic toxicity
Riseman [13]	1990	Case series	17	8	Reduces mortality and need for debridements
Li et al. [14]	2015	Retrospective	16	12	Decreased drainage tube, curative time, and mortality
Schneidewind [15]	2020	Systematic review	145	–	Mortality rate of 16.6% in the HBO group
Mladenov [16]	2022	Retrospective	83	98	High survival in HBOT

Sessions

Most of the studies in the literature as well as our center uses a HBOT protocol of 90 min at 2.0–2.4 ATA 5 days in a week. This can be an aggressive treatment regimen in complex polymicrobial cases with three sessions within 24 h and thereafter twice daily. HBOT sessions are to be given after first and subsequent debridements till cessation of tissue necrosis is achieved. Total sessions can be 10–20 based on clearing infection in the various sessions for different indications and wound becomes viable.

Laboratory Risk Indicator for Necrotizing Infection Score

It was developed in 2004 to indicate severity of infection in NSTI. A score of 8 or greater represents a 75% risk of necrotizing infection.

The parameters of the score are:

1. CRP >150 mg/L.
2. TLC > 25 cells/mm.
3. Hemoglobin<11 g/dl.
4. Sodium<135 mg/dl.
5. Serum creatinine>1.6 mg/dl.
6. Glucose>150 mg/dl.

CT scan helps to give a vivid picture of NSTI. Aspiration and gram stain are done to find the microbiological status of the wound. Ultrasound is of use in confirming subcutaneous gas in affected tissues. Cobblestoning, snow globe effect, and dirty shadowing are ultrasound features seen in Fournier's gangrene.

Fig. 13.4 Post cellulitis
gangrenous changes in
ulnar 3 fingers

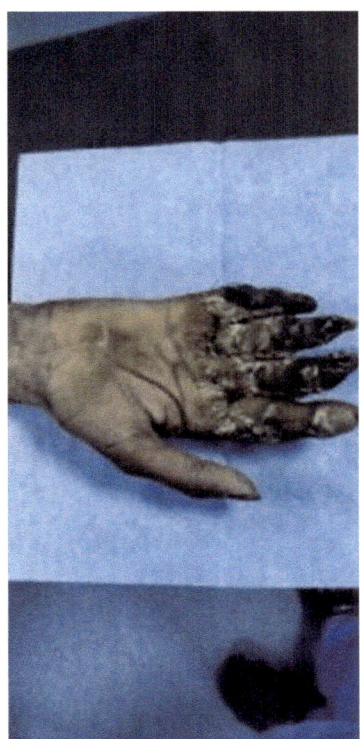

Complications

The various complications encountered are multiorgan failure, septic shock, amputations, and death (Fig. 13.4).

Discussion

A combination of early surgical debridement with suitable antibiotics and hyperbaric therapy improves outcomes of these patients.

HBOT may restore the susceptibility to antibiotics by inducing aerobic metabolism. This has been demonstrated in Pseudomonas aeruginosa and Staphylococcus aureus biofilm models [1]. Oxygen therapy results in detoxification, helpful in cases of intraperitoneal spread, florid septicaemia and where conventional therapy is ineffective [2].

HBOT may interrupt the pathology of NSTI by acting as an intravascular osmotic agent [3].

The incidence of Multi Organ Dysfunction Syndrome was lower in the HBO group than in the non-HBO group hyperbaric oxygen therapy in gas gangrene seems to be life-, limb- and tissue-saving. Early diagnosis remains essential. Patient survival can be improved if the disease is recognized early and appropriate therapy instituted promptly [4]. HBO promotes tissue growth by angiogenesis and inhibit toxin production at high oxygen levels [6]. This study showed killing effect of ciprofloxacin on pseudomonas biofilms is increased by hyperbaric therapy [7]. 16 studies emphasized early initiation of HBO to be useful in cases of maxillofacial necrotising fasciitis with better survival [8]. The authors considered HBO therapy to be optional in maxillofacial cellulitis of head and neck with less mortality [9]. Nine patients of cervical necrotizing fasciitis recieved HBOT showing less debridements and length of stay along with surgical debridement [10].

Six out of 10 (6/10) RCTs reported in this study cited 28 *day mortality* as most common reported time point (40%) of RCTs. *Ninety-day mortality* was more frequently reported in the second five-year period of extraction [11], leading to a mortality rate of 16.6% in the HBO group and 25.9% in the non-HBO group. Meta analysis of data revealed reduced odds of dying in this study with HBOT protocol of 2–2.8ATA for 90 minutes in necrotising soft tissue infections [12]. There was a reduction in mortality and wound morbidity in non clostridial infections with HBO [13]. The number of surgical debridements, drainage catheters and curative time was less in HBOT group treated cases of Fournier gangrene [14]. A systematic review identified 13 relevant studies with 202 cases who recieved HBO showed a low mortality rate of 16.6% in Fournier gangrene cases [15]. Benefit of HBOT is more in critically ill patients and results improve with combining VAC therapy, more debridements and coverage with mesh grafts [16].

Outcomes

Outcomes after HBOT in necrotizing fasciitis favour a decrease in mortality, fewer need of debridements, and improved healing. It plays a beneficial role in patients of Fournier's gangrene by inhibiting and killing anaerobic bacteria. HBOT helps in wound bed preparation by promoting granulation tissue and leads to a better graft uptake (Fig. 13.5). It shortens the hospital stay and improves limb salvage in polymicrobial cases. It improves outcome in high risk cases of cellulitis by reducing inflammation and halts progression.

Fig. 13.5 Improved split thickness graft uptake over right thigh, scrotum and right testis with HBOT sessions

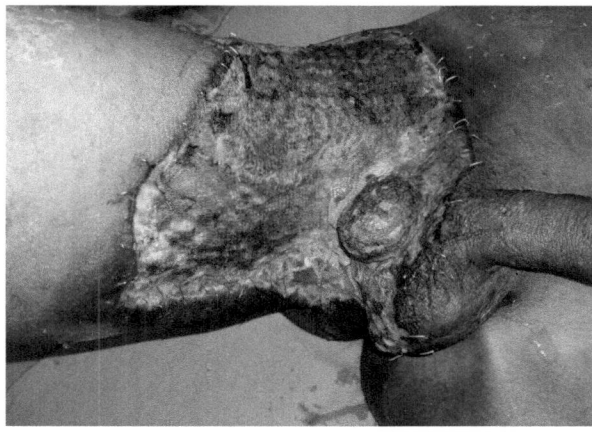

References

1. Lerche CJ, Christophersen LJ, Kolpen M, Nielsen PR, Trøstrup H, Thomsen K, et al. Hyperbaric oxygen therapy augments tobramycin efficacy in experimental Staphylococcus aureus endocarditis. Int J Antimicrob Agents. 2017 50:406–12.
2. Brummelkamp WH, Hogendyk J, Boerema I. Treatment of anaerobic infections by drenching the tissue with oxygen under high atmospheric pressure. Surgery. 1961;49:299–302.
3. Hills BA. A role for oxygen-induced osmosis in hyperbaric oxygen therapy. Med Hypotheses. 1999;52:259–63.
4. Huang C, Zhong Y, Yue C, He B, Li Y, Li J. The effect of hyperbaric oxygen therapy on the clinical outcomes of necrotizing soft tissue infections: a systematic review and meta-analysis. World J Emerg Surg. 2023;18(1):23.
5. Korhonen K. Hyperbaric oxygen therapy in acute necrotizing infections with a special reference to the effects on tissue gas tensions. Ann Chir Gynaecol Suppl. 2000;214:7–36.
6. van Unnika AJM. Inhibition of toxin production in clostridium perfringens in vitro by hyperbaric oxygen. Antonie Van Leeuwenhoek. 1965;31:181–6.
7. Kolpen M, Mousavi N, Sams T, et al. Reinforcement of the bactericidal effect of ciprofloxacin on *Pseudomonas aeruginosa* biofilm by hyperbaric oxygen treatment. Int J Antimicrob Agents. 2016;47:163–7.
8. Kryeziu K, Myftiu B, Hajdari B, Halihajdaraj R, Stubljar D. Efficacity of hyperbaric oxygen therapy for necrotizing fasciitis in the maxillofacial region: The review of the literature. Int Wound J. 2024;21(6):e14915.
9. Thrane JF, Pikelis A, Ovesen T. Hyperbaric oxygen may only be optional in head and neck necrotizing fasciitis: a retrospective analysis of 43 cases and review of the literature. Infect Dis. 2017;49(11–12):792–8.
10. Flanagan CE, Daramola OO, Maisel RH, Adkinson C, Odland RM. Surgical debridement and adjunctive hyperbaric oxygen in cervical necrotizing fasciitis. Otolaryngol Head Neck Surg. 2009;140(5):730–4.
11. Wackett J, Devaney B, Chau R, Ho J, King N, Grewal J, Armstrong J, Mitra B. Reported outcome measures in necrotising soft tissue infections: a systematic review. Diving Hyperb Med. 2024;54(1):47–56.
12. Hedetoft M, Bennett MH, Hyldegaard O. Adjunctive hyperbaric oxygen treatment for necrotising soft-tissue infections: a systematic review and meta-analysis. Diving Hyperb Med. 2021;51(1):34–43.

13. Riseman JA, Zamboni WA, Curtis A, Graham DR, Konrad HR, Ross DS. Hyperbaric oxygen therapy for necrotizing fasciitis reduces mortality and the need for debridements. Surgery. 1990;108:847–50.
14. Li C, Zhou X, Liu LF, Qi F, Chen JB, Zu XB. Hyperbaric oxygen therapy as an adjuvant therapy for comprehensive treatment of Fournier's gangrene. Urol Int. 2015;94:453–8.
15. Schneidewind L, Anheuser P, Schönburg S, Wagenlehner FME, Kranz J. Hyperbaric oxygenation in the treatment of fournier's gangrene: a systematic review. Urol Int. 2021;105(3–4):247–56.
16. Mladenov A, Diehl K, Müller O, et al. Outcome of necrotizing fasciitis and Fournier's gangrene with and without hyperbaric oxygen therapy: a retrospective analysis over 10 years. World J Emerg Surg. 2022;17:43.

Chapter 14
Crush Injury

Introduction

Crush injuries form a major volume of admissions in any tertiary center due to road traffic accidents, industrial mishaps, or natural disasters. Numerous complications can occur in any crush injury of extremities leading to loss of limbs. This incurs a loss of work on the part of the patient, exorbitant costs, and prolonged hospitalization. Crush injury involves a primary injury. i.e., direct impact surrounded by a penumbra of tissues amenable to ongoing ischemia and a zone of secondary injury prone to hypoxia, ischemia, and loss. A hand crush injury involves damage to various hand structures caused by a compressive force, often from high-energy mechanisms like motor vehicle accidents or industrial accidents. This force can damage bones, blood vessels, nerves, and soft tissues, leading to complications like inflammation, swelling, compartment syndrome, and potential tissue necrosis. Open fractures with crush syndrome is associated with infective non-union, osteomyelitis, pain, and disability. Mortality in crush injury increases with age > 50, prior illness, and duration of entrapment.

Etiology of Crush Syndrome

Immobility against firm surface >1 h.
  It is due to:

- Natural disasters—earthquakes, tsunami.
- Man-made disasters—nuclear bombing, explosions.
- Road traffic accidents.
- Industrial mishaps.

V. Mago, *Hyperbaric Medicine*, https://doi.org/10.1007/978-981-95-2644-4_14

It can be due to reduced compartment size following tight dressing or plaster. Compartment size is increased in burns, trauma, ischemia, exercise, combat injuries, and snakebite. Figure 14.1 illustrates gangrene occurring following road traffic crush injury in the right foot.

Crush injuries to the extremities in India, similar to other parts of the world, are often caused by industrial accidents, road traffic incidents, and, in some cases, Earthquakes or cloudbursts. These injuries can lead to a variety of complications, including broken bones, bleeding, bruising, and compartment syndrome. Figure 14.2 shows extent of mutilating crush injury sustained in an industrial accident.

Classification

1. Localized crush injury (Compartment).
    2. Crush syndrome (Systemic).
    3. Specific area—foot/hand/leg.
    4. Severity based—mild/moderate/severe (Figs. 14.1 and 14.2).

Fig. 14.1 Crush injury second and third toes causing gangrene

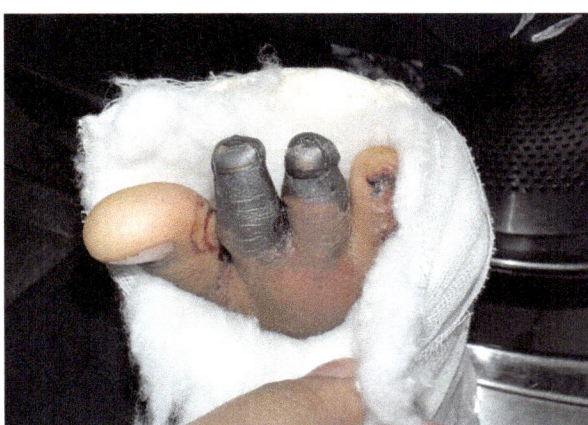

Fig. 14.2 Mutilating hand injury right hand

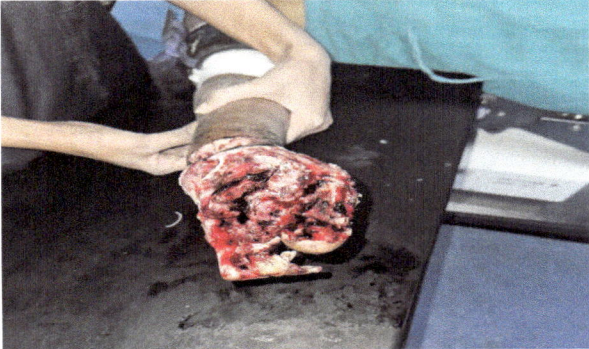

Pathophysiology of Crush Syndrome

Excessive crush or force within 1-6 hours leads to muscle damage and release of toxins. The mechanism of injury is based on the disruption of the triad of ischemia, hypoxia, and edema. The release of toxins from dead muscles leads to myoglobinuria. Compartment syndrome affects the extremities due to third space losses. Hypotension exacerbates renal shutdown. Reperfusion leads to cardiac arrhythmias following imbalance of potassium and calcium due to sudden washout of toxins in systemic circulation. Metabolic acidosis results in renal failure.

Epidemiology

The incidence of crush syndrome is 2–15%. The earthquake victims constitute about 30% and both limbs' involvement is 75%. In India, crush injuries are mostly due to road traffic and industrial accidents. Incidence of compartment is between 2% and 12%. Annual incidence rate is 73.1 per 1000 population. Hand crush injuries are around 40%. Foot crush injuries comprise 7.59% of road traffic accidents.

Evaluation

Clinical examination is important along with a thorough neurovascular status (Fig. 14.2). Routine blood tests and urine examination for myoglobin is needed. ECG is done to look for hyperkalemia. A level of serum creatinine kinase >1000 iU/l is indicator of crush syndrome. Urine output and pH are done hourly and ABG is done every 4 h. Clinically, 5 Ps are pathognomonic of compartment, i.e., pain, pallor, paresthesia, pressure/tension, and pulselessness. Doppler studies are helpful to rule out vascular sequelae. Intercompartment pressure > 30 mmHg indicates need for fasciotomy. X-rays are done to rule out fractures or gas. CT angiography can be done to evaluate the vascular status of extremities.

Effects of HBO

HBO decreases the outflow from the vascular compartment. This reduces edema and promotes wound healing. It reduces anaerobic bacterial growth by its bactericidal effect, and improves immune status. Three HBOT sessions of 2.4 ATA pressure for 90 min are done after fasciotomy. It induces hyperoxygenation and promotes wound healing in a crush injury patient. Patients are treated with HBOT to control compartment pressure in extremities. It reduces muscle necrosis in fasciotomy wounds. It improves survival of tissues in the grey area. Figures 14.3 and 14.4 show the benefits of HBOT in limb salvage. It increases stem cell recruitment, creating

Fig. 14.3 Crush injury
right foot

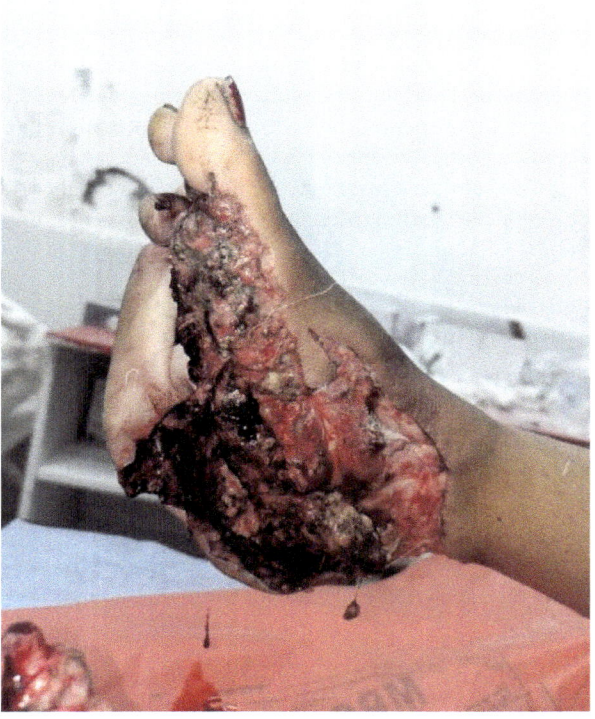

Fig. 14.4 Reduction in
edema and healthy wound
bed after 12 sessions

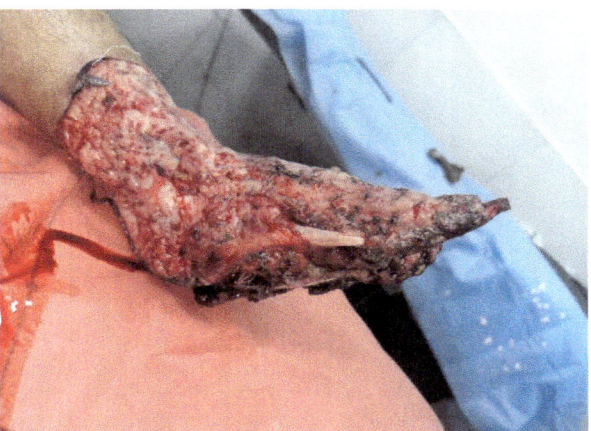

new blood vessels. It mitigates rate of amputation in digits and limbs. This therapy is ant inflammatory, anti oxidant and anti ischemic.

Discussion

Thirty-six patients with crush injuries showed complete healing of wounds after HBOT, especially patients >40 years with grade 3 soft tissue injury [1].

This study emphasizes role of HBOT in reducing tissue necrosis and complications [2]. If first session of HBOT is given <72 h postoperatively, results are better with short length of stay, faster healing, and less number of surgical procedures [3]. The earthquake victims with \MESS score of 7–14 showed improvement in sensory recovery and amputation rates [4].

Aerobic metabolism is accentuated by HBOT in post-ischemia phase [5]. Nitric oxide levels in wound fluid increased after HBOT with a decrease in wound areas of 6 patients at 2 ATA at 4 weeks [6].

Most cases showed an improvement in tissue infection rates with better limb salvage rates in severely mangled extremities [7]. Compartment syndromes involving skeletal muscles respond well with hyperbaric oxygen therapy and prevent complications [8]. Crush injuries were 53% in this study and early HBOT helped in limb salvage and better function after HBOT [9]. Eight out of the 9 studies in this meta-analysis documented a useful role of HBOT in crush injury and traumatic ischemia [10].

Sixteen patients with Gustilo class 3A showed no infections and a reduction in reoperation and adverse effects [11].

Thirty-six patients with crush injuries reported healed wounds and less tissue necrosis [12].

HBOT is beneficial in lower extremity crush injury by improving wound healing, preparing healthy wound bed and early return to work. It improves hypoxia, reverses ischemia, and reduces edema in crush injury.

References

1. Bouachour G, Cronier P, Gouello JP, et al. Hyperbaric oxygen therapy in the management of crush injuries: a randomized double-blind placebocontrolled clinical trial. J Trauma. 1996;41:333–9.
2. Kwee E, Borgdorff M, Schepers T, Halm JA, Winters HAH, Weenink RP, Ridderikhof ML, Giannakópoulos GF. Adjunctive hyperbaric oxygen therapy in the management of severe lower limb soft tissue injuries: a systematic review. Eur J Trauma Emerg Surg. 2024;50(3):1093–100.
3. Chang DH, Hsieh CY, Chang CW, Wang HH, Chang HT. The use of hyperbaric oxygen therapy in the treatment of hand crush injuries. Wound Repair Regen. 2024;32(2):146–54.
4. Demir L, Öztürk M. Use of hyperbaric oxygen therapy in severe earthquake injuries. Ulus Travma Acil Cerrahi Derg. 2024;30(3):185–91.

5. Nylander G, Nordström H, Lewis D, Larsson J. Metabolic effects of hyperbaric oxygen in postischemic muscle. Plast Reconstr Surg. 1987;79(1):91–7.
6. Boykin JV Jr, Baylis C. Hyperbaric oxygen therapy mediates increased nitric oxide production associated with wound healing: a preliminary study. Adv Skin Wound Care. 2007;20(7):382–8.
7. Jirangkul P, Baisopon S, Pandaeng D, Srisawat P. Hyperbaric oxygen adjuvant therapy in severe mangled extremities. Injury. 2021;52(11):3511–5.
8. Strauss MB. The effect of hyperbaric oxygen in crush injuries and skeletal muscle-compartment syndromes. Undersea Hyperb Med. 2012;39(4):847–55.
9. Chiang IH, Tzeng YS, Chang SC. Is hyperbaric oxygen therapy indispensable for saving mutilated hand injuries? Int Wound J. 2017;14(6):929–36.
10. Garcia-Covarrubias L, McSwain NE Jr, Van Meter K, Bell RM. Adjuvant hyperbaric oxygen therapy in the management of crush injury and traumatic ischemia: an evidence-based approach. Am Surg. 2005;71(2):144–51.
11. Yamada N, Toyoda I, Doi T, Kumada K, Kato H, Yoshida S, Shirai K, Kanda N, Ogura S. Hyperbaric oxygenation therapy for crush injuries reduces the risk of complications: research report. Undersea Hyperb Med. 2014;41(4):283–9.
12. Eskes A, Vermeulen H, Lucas C, Ubbink DT. Hyperbaric oxygen therapy for treating acute surgical and traumatic wounds. Cochrane Database Syst Rev. 2013;2013(12):CD008059.

Chapter 15
Hyperbaric Therapy for Avascular Necrosis of the Hip

Introduction

Avascular necrosis or osteonecrosis of the hip is a debilitating condition affecting adults under 50 years of age with a diminished blood supply to the hip as a result of prolonged standing or trivial trauma. The most common symptom reported is severe pain in the hip area, groin, thigh, and buttock. It affects the anterior and superior part of the hip. It can lead to stiffness and alteration of gait in long standing cases. In some patients, rest pain is also seer.. Traumatic osteonecrosis is unilateral, while non-traumatic is bilateral with multifocality.

The cause of this osteonecrosis is trauma, steroids, or alcoholism in the United States; thalassemia in Southeast Asia, and HIV in Africa. The lateral epiphyseal arteries at the femoral neck are most vulnerable to ischemia.

The treatment of avascular necrosis of the femoral head (AVNFH) is by invasive (e.g., core decompression or hip arthroplasty) and, nowadays, non-invasive methods such as hyperbaric oxygen therapy—HBO2 is proving a boon for such patients with alleviation of pain, early weight bearing, and good volume of bone stock.

Epidemiology

In the United States, it is estimated that 300,000–600,000 people have AVN of the hip, with 10,000–20,000 new cases annually. AVN is a leading cause for total hip arthroplasty, accounting for about 10% of cases in the USA. The incidence of AVN varies across different countries and populations. In Korea, it has been reported as 28.9 per 100,000 people, and in India AVN was the indication for 51.8% of primary total hip replacements.

V. Mago, *Hyperbaric Medicine*, https://doi.org/10.1007/978-981-95-2644-4_15

Risk Factors

It can be:

1. Traumatic

    Bone fractures and joint dislocations are predisposing factors. Type of fracture (displaced or undisplaced) and time between injury and surgery are the most critical factors in assessing the risk of developing AVN.

2. Non-traumatic

    Alcohol
    Steroids
    Smoking
    Coagulopathy
    Chemotherapy drugs
    Autoimmune diseases like *Systemic Lupus Erythematosa*, sickle cell

Incidence

AVN is more common in men. The bilateral hips are involved most of the time. Atraumatic AVN presents early in men and children with Legg-Calvé-Perthes are more prone.

Classification

Steinberg classification, which is a modified Ficat, is followed in cases of AVN of the hip.

Stage	Radiograph	MRI
0	Normal	Normal
1	Normal	Abnormal
2	Cystic or sclerosis changes	Abnormal MRI/bone scan
3	Crescent sign	Abnormal MRI/bone scan
4	Flattening femoral head	Abnormal MRI/bone scan
5	Narrowing of joint	Abnormal MRI/bone scan
6	Degenerative changes	Abnormal MRI/bone scan

Evaluation

Diagnosis of AVN can be established based on patients' complaints, medical history, and radiographic findings. Initial evaluation with plain radiographic films demonstrating two orthogonal views is the initial diagnostic standard. Magnetic resonance imaging is recommended for detecting earlier stages of the disease. Computed tomography may be superior to MRI in detecting subchondral fracture.

Methods

A prospective observational study was conducted in our hospital with 77 cases of avascular necrosis of the hip who responded with good results in a multiplace chamber. The inclusion criteria was patients above 18 years age with Stage 1–2 AVN of the hip. Written informed consent was taken from each patient. The patients were given 2.4 ATA for 90 min 5 days in a week.

Results

A notable feature observed in all the patients who received sessions was a decrease in intensity of pain and early weight bearing due to the therapy. A significant amount of improvement was noticed in radiographic examination of the hip performed 3 months later (Fig. 15.1). There was no evidence of articular collapse, and bony sclerosis improved with therapy radiologically.

There was a significant decrease in the marrow edema noticed in both the sequential MRI of patients after 10 cycles of HBOT (Fig. 15.2). A significant decrease in femoral head affection by Modified Kerboul method was noticed as the angle decreased in almost all hips treated. All 77 hips were stage 2 to begin with, out of

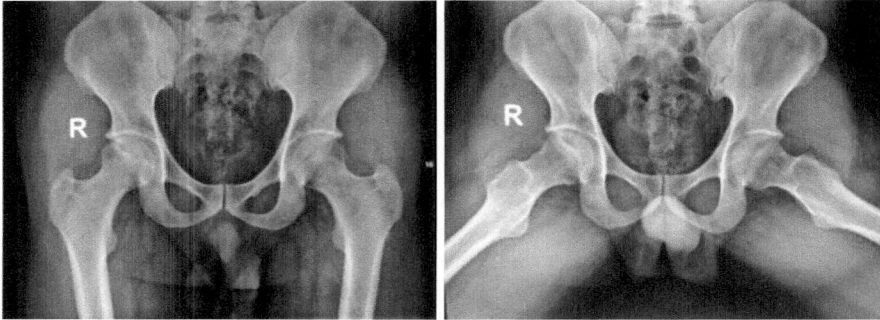

Fig. 15.1 X-ray pelvis showing improvement after 3 months of HBOT

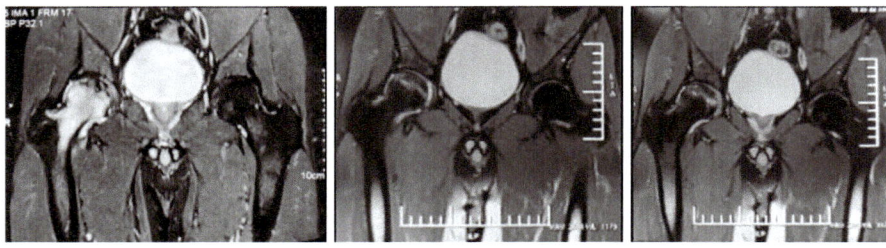

Fig. 15.2 Sequential MRI of patient at pre-HBOT showing areas of marrow surrounded by a low signal intensity rim in hip

Pre HBOT   **Post HBOT**

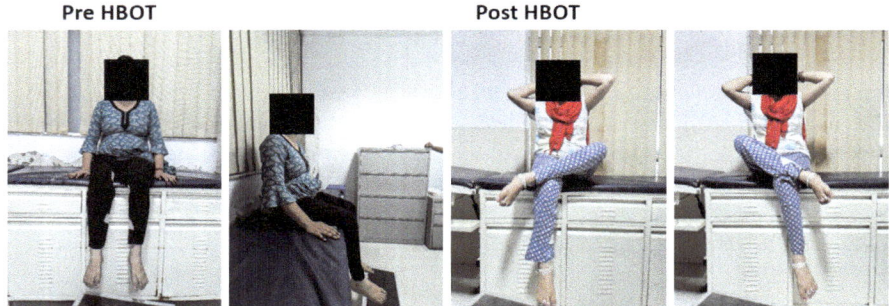

Fig. 15.3 Showing patient able to sit cross-legged after HBOT

Pre HBOT   **Post HBOT**

• Could not
  sit cross
  legged or
  squat due
  to pain

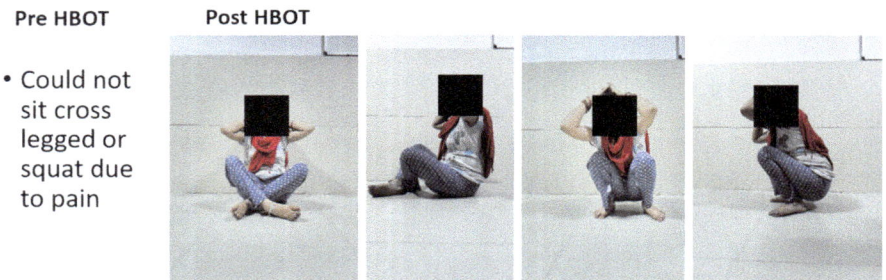

Fig. 15.4 Showing improvement as patient is able to squat and sit cross-legged

which 2 hips improved to ARCO I 3 months after HBOT sessions and a total of 6 hips were ARCO I at 12 months of follow-up.

Patients were able to sit cross-legged and squat after 10 sessions of 2 ATA hyperbaric oxygen therapy administered for 90 min 5 days in a week (Figs. 15.3 and 15.4). The follow-up of patients after 3 months was good and no surgery was needed after a follow-up of 1 year (Fig. 15.5). Hyperbaric oxygen therapy improves the microcirculation, decreases bone edema, and prevents further bone collapse. Treated patients showed improved range of motion of all their hips. HBOT restores oxygen

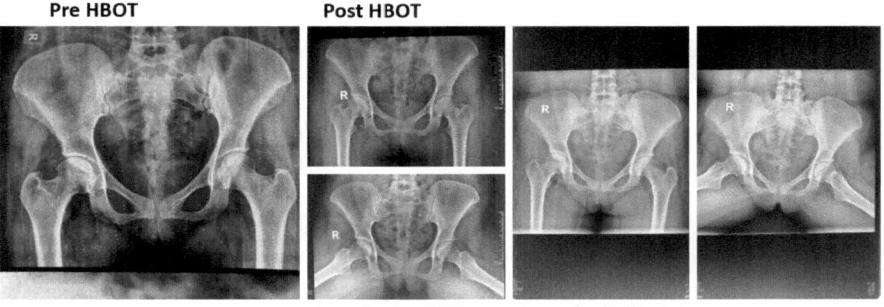

Pre HBOT   **Post HBOT**

3 months after HBOT   1 year after HBOT – Stat. ; quo

Fig. 15.5 Patient showing Radiological recovery at follow-up after one year

supply to ischemic bone, stimulates revascularisation and reduces marrow oedema with marked improvement in pain. Bone repair and remodelling is achieved with angiogenesis, osteogenesis and reperfusion.

Discussion

An early diagnosis, staging, and appropriate management is needed to improve results in femoral head necrosis.

The oxford hip score of 13 patients was 37.3 with improvement in pain scores [1] with hyperbaric therapy. Huang et al. reported a better prognostic index in patients' lesions on MRI based on location and size [2].

Hyperbaric therapy of femoral head group showed improvement in MRI scans in nine of the 14 joints (64%) and after six months 10 joints (71%) had good outcomes [3]. The results of meta-analysis revealed effect of hyperbaric to be 4.95 times higher than control group [4].

Protocols and guidelines have been formulated at the Consensus conference in Lille [5].

The results of this meta-analysis suggest that patients with femoral head necrosis treated with HBO therapy can achieve a significant clinical improvement. In Italy, femoral head necrosis is included in accepted indications supported by reimbursement agencies [6].

The results in this study showed a significant reduction in TNF-α and IL-6 plasma levels over time. This decrease in inflammatory markers mirrored observed reductions in bone marrow edema and reductions in patient self-reported pain in HBOT patients [7].

Twenty-three patients with unilateral ANFH at stages I, II, and III received standard HBOT. Serum OPG levels were obtained at the beginning of HBOT (T0), after 15 sessions (T1), 30 sessions (T2), after a 30-day break (T3), and after 60 sessions (T4). Magnetic resonance imaging (MRI) was obtained at T0 and about 1 year from the end of HBO treatments. Lesion size was compared between pre- and post-HBOT. Nineteen patients completed the study. HBOT reduced pain symptoms in all patients. HBOT significantly reduced lesion size in all stage I and II patients and in 2 of 11 stage-III patients. HBOT increased serum OPG levels, but receptor activator of nuclear factor kappa-B ligand (RANKL) levels did not change [8].

The trial conducted in our hospital emphasized a beneficial role of hyperbaric oxygen therapy in terms of better pain scores, improvement in MRI scans, and better quality of life. Clinical outcomes were remarkable as patients were able to sit cross-legged or squat after therapy with dramatic reduction in pain. With HBOT there is a decreased need for surgery. HBOT improved bone marrow oxygen supply, exerts anti oedema, anti inflammatory effect with induction of osteogenesis in FICAT 1-2 AVN of the hip.

References

1. Salameh M, Moghamis IS, Kokash O, Ahmed GO. Hyperbaric oxygen therapy for the treatment of Steinberg I and II avascular necrosis of the femoral head: a report of fifteen cases and literature review. Int Orthop. 2021;45(10):2519–23.
2. Huang G-S, Chan WP, Chang Y-C, et al. MR imaging of bone marrow edema and joint effusions in patients with osteonecrosis of the femoral head: relationship to pain. AJR. 2003;181:545–9.
3. Currie JR, Gawthrope IC, Banham ND. The use of hyperbaric oxygen for avascular necrosis of the femoral head and femoral condyle: a single center's experience over 30 years. Diving Hyperb Med. 2024;54(2):92–6.
4. Li W, Ye Z, Wang W, Wang K, Li L, Zhao D. Clinical effect of hyperbaric oxygen therapy in the treatment of femoral head necrosis: a systematic review and meta-analysis. Orthopedics. 2017;46(5):440–6.
5. Camporesi E, Vezzani G, Zanon V, Manelli D, Enten G, Quartesan S, Bosco G. Review on hyperbaric oxygen treatment in femoral head necrosis. Undersea Hyperb Med. 2017;44(6):497–508.
6. Paderno E, Zanon V, Vezzani G, Giacon TA, Bernasek TL, Camporesi EM, Bosco G. Evidence-supported HBO therapy in femoral head necrosis: a systematic review and meta-analysis. Int J Environ Res Public Health. 2021;18(6):2888.
7. Bosco G, Vezzani G, Sposta SM, Rizzato A, Enten G, Abou-Samra A, Malacrida S, Quartesan S, Vezzoli A, Camporesi E. Hyperbaric oxygen therapy ameliorates osteonecrosis in patients by modulating inflammation and oxidative stress. J Enzym Inhib Med Chem. 2018;33:1501–5.
8. Vezzani G, Quartesan S, Cancellara P, Camporesi E, Mangar D, Bernasek T, Dalvi P, Yang Z, Paoli A, Rizzato A, Bosco G. Hyperbaric oxygen therapy modulates serum OPG/RANKL in femoral head necrosis patients. J Enzyme Inhib Med Chem. 2017;32(1):707–11.

Chapter 16
Central Retinal Artery Occlusion

Introduction

CRAO is an ophthalmic emergency. Incidence is 1 in 100,000 patients. This disease leads to sudden painless loss of vision and peripheral fields. The blockade can be at the level of central retinal artery or branch retinal artery or cilioretinal artery. Poor prognosis of the visual acuity is due to lack of effective treatment modalities. Hyperbaric improves the circulation of retina by hyperoxygenation and preserves outer retinal wall thickness. CRVO-related CRAO should be regarded as a rare complication of exposure to high altitudes. Certain risk factors increase the propensity to cause occlusion, especially in males and those with unilateral carotid artery stenosis.

Risk Factors

Hypertension
Diabetes
Hyperlipidemia
High BMI
Hypercoagulable states
Cardiac diseases

V. Mago, *Hyperbaric Medicine*, https://doi.org/10.1007/978-981-95-2644-4_16

Anatomy and Pathophysiology

The central retinal artery enters the globe 1 cm behind it. It supplies watershed zone between 2 vascular systems supplied by central retinal and short posterior ciliary artery. Inner retina loses its vascular supply due to blockade of central retinal artery by an embolus. The embolus can be cholesterol (most common), platelet fibrin, or calcified. Retinal ganglion cell infarction occurs due to this blockade. The retina is opacified and white as a result, cherry red spot is seen on fundoscopy due to preserved choroidal circulation.

Types of CRAO

Arteritic—seen in old people with scalp tenderness and jaw pain especially in cases
   of giant cell arteritis, worst prognosis.
Non-arteritic—spares cilioretinal artery.
Staging of CRAO.
Incomplete—low visual acuity, delayed flow, mild edema in retina.
Subtotal—decreased visual acuity, cherry red spot.
Complete—No light perception and no blood flow.

Mechanism of Action

HBOT has been found to be useful by increasing oxygenation of choroidal vessels and adding oxygen to vitreous body which acts as a reservoir maintaining supply of the retina. This therapy increases the thickness of choroidal vessels. The thickness of outer retinal layer increases with therapy as shown in many clinical trials.

Dose of HBO

The treatment should be started once the diagnosis is made and a pressure of 2 ATA is given for 90 min for 3 days twice daily. If there is no improvement in vision, pressure is raised to 2.4 ATA for 90 min.

Discussion

Hyperbaric plays an important role in restoring visual acuity in non-arteritic cases.
   The authors outlined the protocol of HBOT in CRAO cases where 2 ATA pressure was given for 90 min with good results [1].

Seven RCTs outlined in this meta-analysis have shown importance and benefit of HBOT in central retinal artery occlusion if therapy is given for more than 9 h [2]. Patients with CRAO who were treated within a timeline of 9 h gave early return of visual acuity [3]. Enhanced depth imaging optical coherence tomography parameters in this trial showed an increase in central fovea and outer retinal layer thickness with improved visual acuity [4]. The authors found, in a cohort of 63 patients of CRAO, 3 patterns of manifestations—poor flow, exudation, and mixed types in fluorescein angiography of the fundus [5]. Emergency HBOT plays a vital role in restoration of vision if instituted within first 72 h [6].

Oxygen as a drug, if provided early in CRAO, restores vision due to hyperoxygenation of choroidal vessels and prevents irreversible effects on the retina.

References

1. Celebi ARC. Hyperbaric oxygen therapy for central retinal artery occlusion: patient selection and perspectives. Clin Ophthalmol. 2021;15:3443–57.
2. Wu X, Chen S, Li S, et al. Oxygen therapy in patients with retinal artery occlusion: a meta-analysis. PLoS One. 2018;13(8):e0202154.
3. Kim BM, Wang KY, Xu TT, Hooshmand SJ, Toups GN, Millman MP, Steinkraus LW, Tooley AA, Barkmeier AJ, Chen JJ. Outcomes of hyperbaric oxygen treatment for central retinal artery occlusion: a single center experience. Am J Ophthalmol. 2025;269:393–401.
4. Lee JM, Choi SH, Jeon GS, Chang IB, Wang SJ, Hong IH. A comprehensive evaluation of efficacy of hyperbaric oxygen therapy in non-arteritic central retinal artery occlusion using enhanced depth imaging optical coherence tomography. Sci Rep. 2024;14(1):23676.
5. Gong H, Song Q, Wang L. Manifestations of central retinal artery occlusion revealed by fundus fluorescein angiography are associated with the degree of visual loss. Exp Ther Med. 2016;11(6):2420–4.
6. Murphy-Lavoie H, Butler F, Hagan C. Central retinal artery occlusion treated with oxygen: a literature review and treatment algorithm. Undersea Hyperb Med. 2012;39(5):943–53.

Chapter 17
Hyperbaric in Idiopathic Sensorineural Hearing Loss

Introduction

Idiopathic sudden sensorineural hearing loss (ISSHL) is considered an otolaryngologic emergency. It is diagnosed by the triad of hearing loss of 30 dB over 3 successive frequencies for 3 days. The incidence of SSNHL is 5–20 per 100,000 with about 66,000 new cases in the USA per year. It affects 7.9–13.3% of the Indian population. Hearing function in the inner ear is maintained by the cochlea which is known to have a high oxygen demand. Cochlear hypoxia is associated with progressive ossification, fibrosis, loss of neurons, endolymphatic hydrops, and hearing loss. Direct blood supply to the organ of Corti is minimal; oxygen must diffuse through the perilymph and cortilymph. The labyrinthine artery (internal auditory artery) is a long, slender branch-off of the anterior inferior cerebellar artery (85%) or the basilar artery (15%).

In developed countries, approximately 80% of congenital hearing impairment has a genetic origin. The two most common bacterial infections known to cause SSNHL in the United States are Lyme disease and syphilis. It typically occurs between 43 years and 53 years of age, with equal sex distribution. The etiology can be infectious, autoimmune, traumatic, vascular, neoplastic, metabolic (diabetes), and neurologic (pontine ischemia).

The most common syndromic form of hereditary sensorineural hearing loss, Pendred syndrome, is inherited in an autosomal-recessive fashion.

V. Mago, *Hyperbaric Medicine*, https://doi.org/10.1007/978-981-95-2644-4_17

Classification

1. Based on cause:
   • Genetic.
   • Environmental.
   • Multifactorial.
2. Time of onset:
   • Congenital/acquired.
3. Age—prelingual/postlingual.
4. linical:
   • Non syndromic.
   • Syndromic—Pendred, Jarvell Lange Nielsen, Stickler, Waardenburg.
5. Frequency—low/mid/high.
6. Ears involved—unilateral/bilateral.
7. Degree of hearing loss:
   • Mild—26–40 dB.
   • Moderate—41–55 dB.
   • Severe—71–90 dB.
   • Profound— > 90 dB.

Clinical Features

The symptoms are tinnitus, dizziness, hearing loss in one ear and unable to understand speech (sounds like s or h). The TV seems loud to some patients and others think you are mumbling words. Most of the cases are unilateral and 2% have bilateral involvement. Aural fullness is seen in 15% cases.

Diagnosis

Otoscopy is done to rule out wax. The Weber and Rinne tests are performed using a 512 Hz tuning fork where sound is lateralized to good ear and air conduction lasts longer than bone conduction. Hearing acuity is measured by ABR, tympanometry, and OAE estimation. Clinicians should evaluate patients with sudden sensorineural hearing loss for retrocochlear pathology by obtaining magnetic resonance imaging or auditory brainstem response. An SNHL of greater than 90 dB in all frequencies was considered a profound loss. CT scans are useful to diagnose large vestibular aqueduct or cochlear dysplasia. Genetic evaluation with ophthalmology check-up is mandatory in syndromic cases of hearing loss.

HBOT Therapy

Schedule of Sessions

The American Academy of Otolaryngology recommends hyperbaric as a treatment option for up to 3 months after symptom onset. Treatment pressure for hyperbaric oxygen therapy should be 2.0 ATA to 2.4 ATA for 90 min daily for 10–20 treatments depending on the response. Treatment sessions with above protocol has shown improvement in 2 patients with 50% improvement in a cohort of 6 patients in our hospital.

The optimal time for treatment is within 2 weeks of onset, as delaying treatment can greatly decrease its efficacy. The benefits of hyperbaric are:

- Increase the oxygenation of the inner ear and rapidly corrects the hypoxia of the inner ear.
- It increases the oxygen partial pressure of the perilymphatic fluid.
- It alleviates cochlear damage caused by ischemia-reperfusion and free radicals.
- It reduces the occurrence of inflammation mediated by various inflammatory mediators such as reactive oxygen species.
- It promotes vasoconstriction to reduce edema.

Scuba diving is prohibited after therapy because of the associated risk of ear injuries. Adequate noise protection is used. Prognosis for recovery is less in female patients, with descending patterns of hearing loss, coexistence of vertigo, and older age.

Discussion

Hyperbaric oxygen therapy (HBOT) has been a treatment for ISSNHL in the late 1970s, but it has only recently been widely used in China. The efficacy of corticosteroid therapy for sudden sensorineural hearing loss remains unproven. Studies have reported that HBOT can effectively alleviate symptoms and improve curative effects. HBOT effectively alleviates inner ear edema, improves blood circulation, and suppresses inflammation and plays an important role in the treatment of idiopathic sudden sensorineural hearing loss.

The therapeutic window can be missed in treating these cases as cochlear cells are non regenerative [1]. 20 HBOT sessions were useful to bring relief in 178 cases which had early onset and low hearing losses [2]. Twelve of 21 cases (57.14%) of complete hearing loss showed recovery [3].

Hyperbaric oxygen therapy resulted in hearing improvement in 80% of patients: 39% had hearing improvement and 41% had full recovery [4]. Bagli recommended HBO2 therapy in the early period, particularly within 14 days of onset [5]. Hearing thresholds were significantly lower after HBOT compared to pre-treatment values across all patients with a median value of recovery of 22.5 dB [6].

The benefit of HBOT in 1201 patients was greater in groups with severe hearing loss at baseline, HBOT as a salvage treatment [6].

Absolute hearing gain was significantly greater in the HBOT + MT group.

The patients with pure tone average less than 81 dB who were younger than 60 years had better response to HBO treatment than those with profound deafness and in the elderly [7].

This study emphasized the role of steroids with 10 treatments of hyperbaric oxygen therapy to benefit more as compared to >10 treatments [8]. At 6 weeks post treatment, 22% (32/144) had normal hearing (PTA4 < 25 dB), and 69% (99/144) had a PTA4 gain $\geq$10 dB.

This study found severe hearing loss treatment with HBO2 improves by 37.7 dB, 19.3 dB for those with moderate loss, and 15.6 dB improvement overall [9].

The authors proposed the use of 2.5 ATA pressure was more efficient at low frequency losses. The higher frequency losses responded to 2.0 ATA pressure [10]. Patients with severe hearing loss responded more with early HBOT [11], especially those with low frequency descending audiogram and steroid use.

Clinicians have the option to offer hyperbaric oxygen therapy combined with steroid therapy within 2 weeks of onset of sudden sensorineural hearing loss according to clinical practice guidelines (KAS 9b) [12].

Hyperbaric oxygen is used as a supplement to first line therapy in the management of refractory sensorineural hearing loss. Early treatment is advocated in severe cases preferably within 14 days of onset.

References

1. Hu Y, Ye Y, Ji X, Wu J. The role of hyperbaric oxygen in idiopathic sudden sensorineural hearing loss. Med Gas Res. 2024;14(4):180–5.
2. Xie S, Qiang Q, Mei L, et al. Multivariate analysis of prognostic factors for idiopathic sudden sensorineural hearing loss treated with adjuvant hyperbaric oxygen therapy. Eur Arch Otorrinolaringol. 2018;275:47–51.
3. Wang Y, Gao Y, Wang B, Chen L, Zhang X. Efficacy and prognostic factors of combined hyperbaric oxygen therapy in patients with idiopathic sudden sensorineural hearing loss. Am J Audiol. 2019;28(1):95–100.
4. Van Der Wal AW, Van Ooij PJ, De Ru JA. Hyperbaric oxygen therapy for sudden sensorineural hearing loss in divers. J Laryngol Otol. 2016;130(11):1039–47.
5. Bagli BS. Clinical efficacy of hyperbaric oxygen therapy on idiopathic sudden sensorineural hearing loss. Undersea Hyperb Med. 2020;47:51–6.
6. Rhee TM, Hwang D, Lee JS, Park J, Lee JM. Addition of hyperbaric oxygen therapy vs medical therapy alone for idiopathic sudden sensorineural hearing loss: a systematic review and meta-analysis. JAMA Otolaryngol Head Neck Surg. 2018;144(12):1153–61.
7. Cvorovic L, Jovanovic MB, Milutinovic Z, Arsovic N, Djeric D. Randomized prospective trial of hyperbaric oxygen therapy and intratympanic steroid injection as salvage treatment of sudden sensorineural hearing loss. Otol Neurotol. 2013;34(6):1021–6.

8. Laupland BR, Laupland KB, Thistlethwaite K. Hyperbaric oxygen therapy for idiopathic sudden sensorineural hearing loss: a cohort study of 10 versus more than 10 treatments. Diving Hyperb Med. 2024;54(4):275–80.
9. LeGros TL, Murphy-Lavoie H. HBO2 for sudden sensorineural hearing loss. Undersea Hyperb Med. 2020;47(2):271–95.
10. Krajcovicova Z, Melus V, Zigo R, Matisakova I, Vecera J, Kralova E. Hyperbaric oxygen therapy in treatment of sudden sensorineural hearing loss: finding for the maximal therapeutic benefit of different applied pressures. Undersea Hyperb Med. 2019;46(5):665–72.
11. Korpinar S, Alkan Z, Yigit O, Gör A, Toklu A, Cakir B, et al. Factors influencing the outcome of idiopathic sudden sensorineural hearing loss treated with hyperbaric oxygen therapy. Eur Arch Otorrinolaringol. 2011;268:41–7.
12. Chandrasekhar SS, Tsai Do BS, Schwartz SR, et al. Clinical practice guideline: sudden hearing loss (update). Otolaryngol Head Neck Surg. 2019.161(1 suppl):S1–S45.

.

Chapter 18
Gas Gangrene

Introduction

This fulminating infection induces toxins to release gas inducing tissue death. It affects arms and legs. It is treated as a medical emergency. Tissues at high risk of causing gas gangrene are deep wounds, muscle trauma, crushed tissues contaminated with soil or dirt. Predisposing conditions in gas gangrene are diabetes, frost bite, colon cancer, atherosclerosis, and open vessel disease. It is a rapidly fatal disorder resulting in death. Fournier's is vascular infective gangrene of scrotum with obliterative arteritis.1.3% of cases of road traffic accidents lead to gas gangrene.

Types of Gangrene (clinical)

Dry—commonly limbs/arterial obstruction, Figs. 18.1 and 18.2 show defects due to gangrene of soft tissues. A line of demarcation is present. Arterial occlusion is seen.

Wet—more common in bowel/venous obstruction and in cases of bed sores or diabetes. No line of demarcation with venous obstruction.

Gas gangrene—Involves limbs. A type of wet gangrene with gas and myonecrosis caused by clostridia

Internal gangrene—Seen in appendix or bowel loops or untreated hernias.

Fournier gangrene—involves scrotum or groin or perineum.

Fig. 18.1 Gangrene involving avulsed flap following trauma

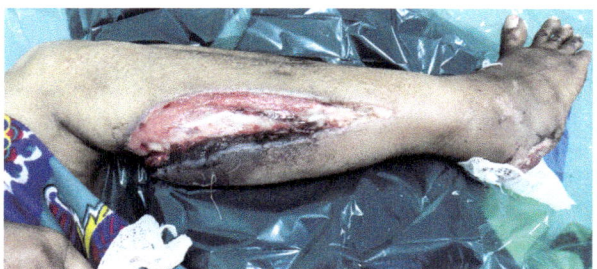

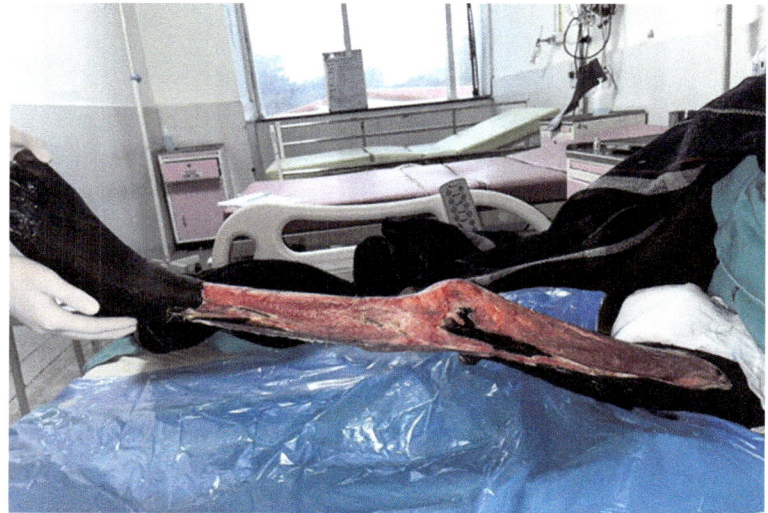

Fig. 18.2 Post NSTI wound left thigh and leg with necrosed tendons

Types of Gas Gangrene

Fulminant, massive, subcutaneous, single.

Toxin Classification

Alpha—lecithinase, attacks sphingomyelin, hemolytic.
Beta toxin—neurotoxic.
Theta toxin—targets RBC, potent cytolysin.
Epsilon toxin—enterocolitis.
Iota—Induces necrosis, apoptosis.
Lambda—targets RBC, WBC, platelets.
Kappa toxins—collagenase, gelatinase.

Epidemiology

In the USA, around 3000 cases are seen. The global incidence of gas gangrene is 0.1–1 case per 100000 population per year. O.1–2% cases of trauma become infected. In India an exponential growth of gas gangrene cases were seen from 12.9% to 40% and 30% of Fournier's gangrene cases were reported from Coimbatore.

Etiology

It is caused by gram positive anaerobic spore-bearing bacilli. It is caused by:

Clostridium perfringens—Gram positive, non motile, spore bearing, capsulated-Most common
Clostridium septicum—non trumatic cases
Clostridium oedematiens—hematogenous spread by GI tract
Clostridium histolyticum—collagenase producer

Source of infection is manured soil and normal intestines. Non-clostridial causes such as coliforms are also seen. It is seen in immunocompromised patients, hematologic malignancies, diabetes and bowel ischemia.

Pathophysiology

A focus of recent injury or wound is invaded by anaerobic bacteria leading to its growth and multiplication. Formation of gas and toxins ensues with damage to tissues, blood vessels, and cells.

Spores enter devitalized tissue and start germinating, leading to multiplication of bacteria. These bacteria release exotoxins causing local muscle damage and systemic multiorgan failure.

Clinical Features

Swelling and pain of the arms or legs are seen. Pale skin with blister formation is seen with formation of gas under the tissues. A crackly sensation is felt over the skin. Sickly sweet odor is perceived with a khaki colored skin due to hemolysis.

Evaluation

A thorough physical examination is mandatory. Blood, fluid, and tissue cultures are done for documenting Clostridium perfringens. The imaging studies like MRI, CT, and X-rays are done to reveal gas in tissues. Duplex scan is done to rule out arterial or venous obstruction. Toxin assays are done. PCR tests are done for rapid detection of clostridial DNA.

Effects and Dose of HBOT

Treatment of gas gangrene is instituted by giving 3 ATA pressure of 100% oxygen for 90 min three times in first 24 h. This is followed by twice daily for 5 days. This treatment is tailored with response achieved. Figures 18.3 and 18.4 show the importance of HBOT therapy in management of post-trauma infected ulcers with gangrene with healing of ulcers noted after 10 sessions. Neutrophil oxidative burst is initiated by high oxygen content. The toxins are neutralized with high oxygen tensions delivered by HBOT. HBOT reduces mortality in synergism with debridements. It decreases the rate of amputations in diabetic foot ulcers. It improves effectiveness of imipenem, aminoglycosides and beta lactams in hypoxic tissues.

Anti-infective effects of HBO

- HBOT is bacteriostatic or batericidal in its efficacy.
- It has synergistic effect with aminoglycosides, imipenem, or ciprofloxacin antibiotics.
- It regulates host defense mechanisms by reducing oedema.

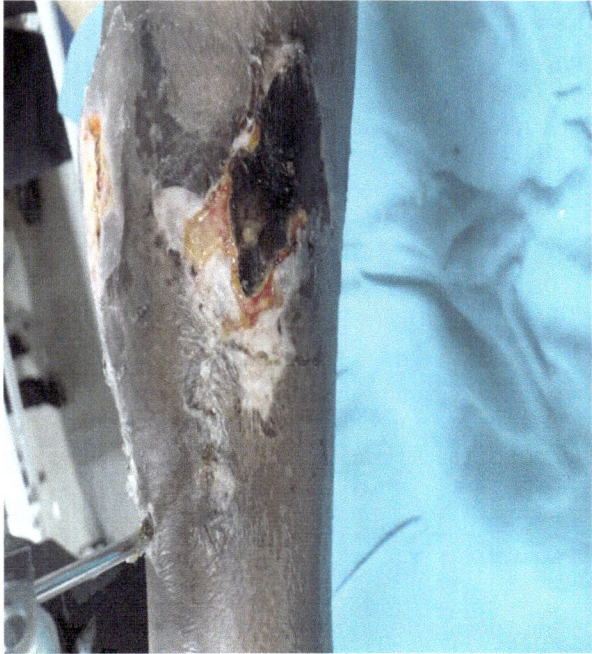

Fig. 18.3 Post-trauma skin gangrene compound fracture right tibia with External fixator

Fig. 18.4 Post-HBOT 10 sessions with healed ulcer

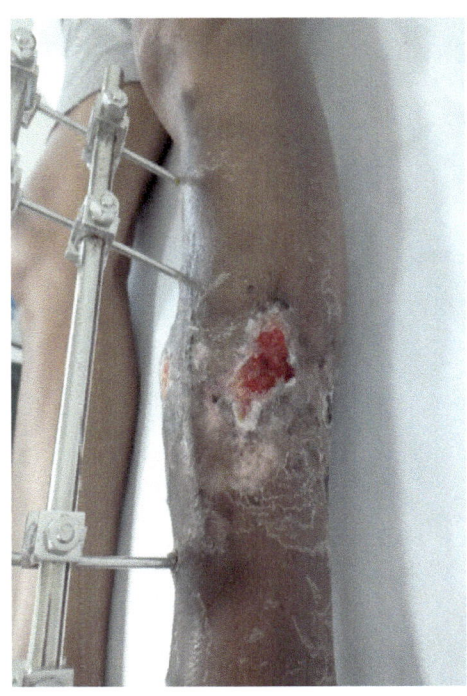

Fig. 18.5 Gangrenous changes at periphery of avulsed flap in trauma case

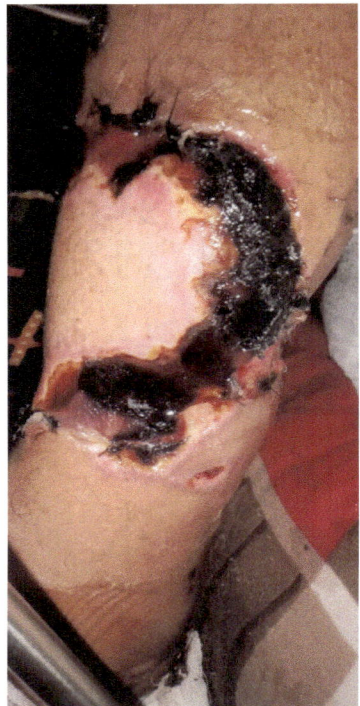

Fig. 18.6 Post
debridement and 5 sessions
of HBOT with
improvement in wound bed

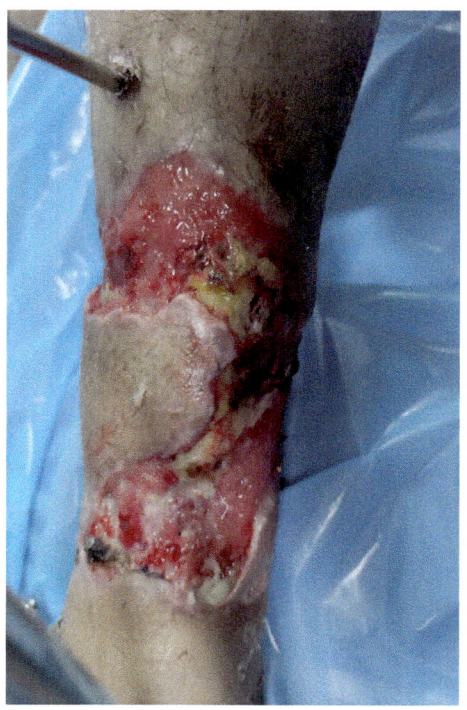

Hyperbaric therapy demarcates viable from non-viable tissue and leads to toxin eradication within 24 h along with antibiotics and debridements. Reactive oxygen species are activated in the wounds which destroy toxins. Figures 18.5 and 18.6 show the benefit of HBOT in gangrenous changes noted at periphery of flaps which, after debridement, develop a demarcation with viable tissue and subsequent sessions improve wound bed preparation. HBOT improves survival of amputation stumps with debridement and 10 sessions of HBOT come out with good results (Figs. 18.7 and 18.8).

Fig. 18.7 Amputation stump right knee with gangrenous muscle and necrotic tissue

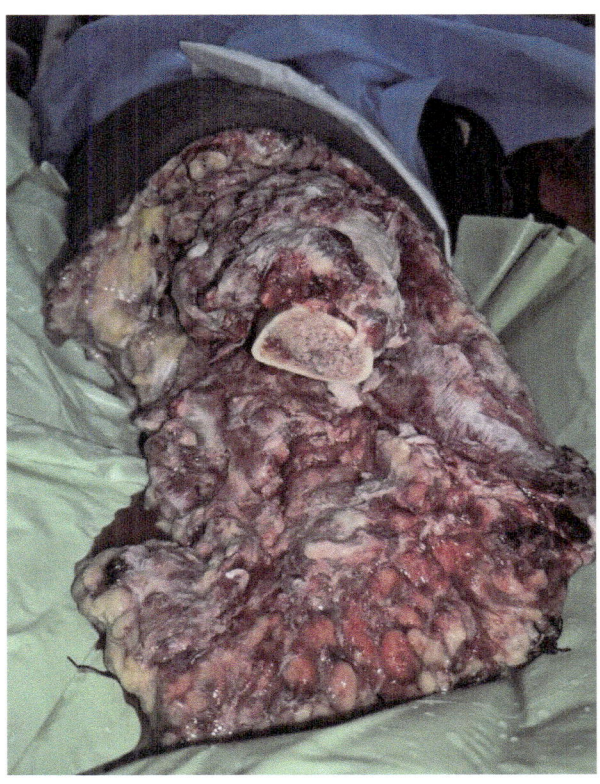

Fig. 18.8 Improvement in wound bed after debridement and HBOT 10 sessions

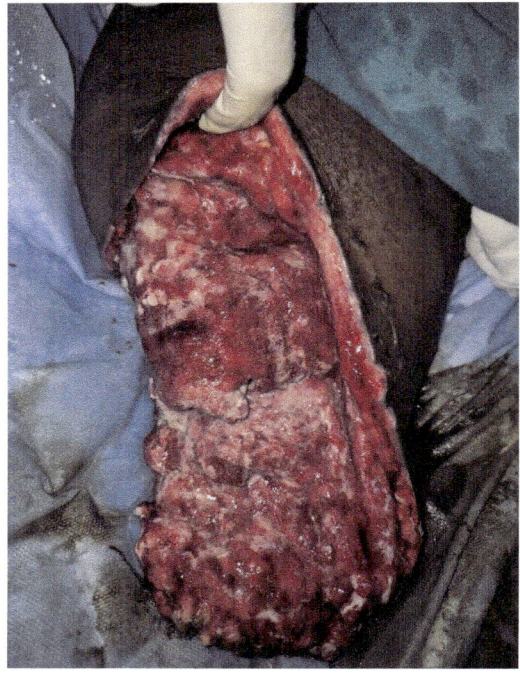

Discussion

Eleven out of 17 cases of gas gangrene survived with HBOT [1]. Three out of 77 patients died in this study with Fournier's gangrene as compared to 34/118 in non-HBOT, outlining reduced mortality [2]. Myocardial infarction was the most common complication in 26 patients of Fournier's treated with HBOT [3]. HBOT group reported less number of debridements, drainage tubes, and low mortality [4].

Hyperbaric oxygen at 3 ATA cured 26 cases of clostridial gas gangrene even with intraperitoneal spread [5]. Thirty-two patients of clostridial myositis treated with HBOT had complete wound healing and patients were able to walk home [6]. The authors described 2 main types of gas gangrene, i.e., traumatic and spontaneous [7]. HBOT decreased infection rates, systemic toxicity in 42 patients of gas gangrene subjected to 2.5 ATA [8].

HBOT improves the delivery of oxygen in devitalized tissue and exerts an anti-infective effect with destruction of toxins, propagating wound healing. Early initiation improves results with better outcomes by reducing spread of necrosis and toxin mediated damage.

References

1. Hirn M, Niinikoski J. Hyperbaric oxygen in the treatment of clostridial gas gangrene. Ann Chir Gynaecol. 1988;77(1):37–40.
2. Feres O, Feitosa MR, Ribeiro da Rocha JJ, Miranda JM, Dos Santos LE, Féres AC, et al. Hyperbaric oxygen therapy decreases mortality due to Fournier's gangrene: a retrospective comparative study. Med Gas Res. 2021;11:18–23.
3. Mindrup SR, Kealey GP, Fallon B. Hyperbaric oxygen for the treatment of fournier's gangrene. J Urol. 2005 Jun;173(6):1975–7.
4. Li C, Zhou X, Liu LF, Qi F, Chen JB, Zu XB. Hyperbaric oxygen therapy as an adjuvant therapy for comprehensive treatment of Fournier's gangrene. Urol Int. 2015;94(4):453–8.
5. Brummelkamp WH, Boerema I, Hoogendyk L. Treatment of clostridial infections with hyperbaric oxygen drenching. A report on 26 cases. Lancet. 1963;1(7275):235–8.
6. Hirn M. Hyperbaric oxygen in the treatment of gas gangrene and perineal necrotizing fasciitis. A clinical and experimental study. Eur J Surg Suppl. 1993;570:1–36.
7. Hussain H, Fadel A, Garcia E, Hernandez RJ, Saadoon ZF, Naseer L, Casmartino E, Hamad M, Schnepp T, Sarfraz R, Angly S, Jayakumar AR. Clostridial myonecrosis: a comprehensive review of toxin pathophysiology and management strategies. Microorganisms. 2024;12(7):1464.
8. Korhonen K, Klossner J, Hirn M, Niinikoski J. Management of clostridial gas gangrene and the role of hyperbaric oxygen. Ann Chir Gynaecol. 1999;88(2):139–42.

Chapter 19
Decompression Sickness

Introduction

Pressure-related injuries arise in a variety of scenarios like diving, compressed-air construction work (e.g., Caisson disease), work in hyperbaric chambers, and being in disabled submarines. There is a reduction in pressure which results in dissolved nitrogen coming out of solution and expanding as bubbles in veins and tissues, the injury often referred to as decompression sickness (DCS) or "the bends." Half a million to four million people in the United States participate in recreational diving. Air embolism can occur after insertion of hemodialysis catheter or intervention radiology procedures. It can occur in breath hold divers referred to as "Taravana."

DCI is a great imitator and affects various organ systems masquerading as:

1. Musculoskeletal pain—most common symptom in altitude-induced DCI.
2. Neurologic(bends) as headache and paresthesia.
3. Dermatologic rash—due to bubbles in dermis.
4. Respiratory (chokes).
5. Spinal cord (hits).
6. Ear (staggers).

Types of DCS:

A. Type 1—Milder variety with mottling, lymphoedema, or musculoskeletal pain.
B. Type 2—It is more severe with inner ear involvement (staggers), lungs (chokes), and the CNS.
C. Type 3—Fatal pulmonary complications like arterial gas embolism.

Most cases of altitude-based DCI occur as low as at 8000 feet and risks increase at higher altitudes. The risk factors of altitude-based sickness are related to:

1. Increased duration.
2. Increased repetition.

V. Mago, *Hyperbaric Medicine*, https://doi.org/10.1007/978-981-95-2644-4_19

3. Increased activity at altitude.
4. Failure to use oxygen.

DCS is caused by the formation of and an increase in the size of extravascular and intravascular bubbles when the sum of the dissolved gas tensions (i.e., oxygen, carbon dioxide, nitrogen, and helium) and when water vapor exceeds the local absolute pressure.

Acute mountain sickness is the negative effect of high altitude due to low oxygen levels. It also occurs in people who work in tunnels or to astronauts.

Classification of diving emergencies are:

• Injuries of the surface.
• Injuries during descent—barotrauma.
• Injuries at the bottom—nitrogen narcosis.
• Injuries during ascent—decompression illness, pulmonary overpressure.

Pathophysiology

Nitrogen reaches equilibrium in tissues slowly particularly in the fat compartment, therefore women and the obese are at a higher risk. A no decompression limit of a diver is maximum time a diver can spend at a depth without requiring decompression stops. It is based on how much nitrogen a diver's body absorbs over a duration of time. At 10 m depth, decompression risk is low and density is doubled. At 33 feet, pressure becomes 2 ATA, volume is half and density is doubled. The dive tables are like your underwater roadmap. Pressure changes faster in ocean diving. If a diver exceeds the depth, ascent should be slow to allow dissolved nitrogen to escape out of the lungs. Exercise before dive or decompression does not increase the number of bubbles. Gas formation occurs in tight tendons causing bends. Bubble induce changes in cell membrane permeability leading to hypovolemia. Bubbles can be seen in anterior chamber of the eye or in CSF. Bubbles trapped in the lungs lead to chokes and a state of non-cardiogenic pulmonary edema. Increase in volume of gas trapped in the lungs leads to alveolar rupture. The gas may extravasate to cause mediastinal emphysema. This is seen in amateur divers. Nucleation of the white matter can result.

Fat emboli damage the blood–brain barrier and cause cerebral edema. Low oxygen content in venous blood is exaggerated by emboli leading to demyelination and axonal damage in the brain. Bubbles are seen in the myelin sheath at high pressures.

Increased altitude increases respiratory rate, blood pH, and increase in urination rate. Acclimatization to high altitude increases RBC production and increased ability to use oxygen.

Increased activity during pressure change increases risk of DCI by formation of gas microemboli by rapid flow of blood, increased local CO_2 production and reduced solubility of gas due to high core temperature.

The nitrogen bubbles lead to:

1. Inflammation at gas tissue interface.
2. Ischemia due to blood flow obstruction.
3. Coagulation at gas blood interface.
4. Emboli cause obstruction and damage structures compressing nearby structures.

Depth intoxication is a result of breathing compressed inert gas. Nitrogen is the gas responsible for CNS effects. Venous emboli form in deep dives or rapid exposure to altitude. Patent PFO increases DCI in brain, spinal cord, and ears. Intravascular bubbles lead to plasma leak and hypovolemia. Injury to pulmonary capillaries leads to pulmonary edema.

Vacuum phenomenon is recognized in radiologic studies where an enclosed tissue space expands in a rebound phenomenon after an external impact. Pressure within the space decreases to decrease solubility of gases. This allows gases to leave a solution. This phenomenon is accelerated after diving and during decompression.

Epidemiology

According to DAN, fewer than 1% of divers experience decompression sickness (DCS). DCS risk is higher in males. The water pressure increases by 1 ATM for every 10 m (33 ft) of seawater and for every 10.4 m (34 ft) of freshwater. The greater the supersaturation, the greater the likelihood that symptomatic DCS will occur. The DCS incidence rate in commercial decompression diving has been reported to be as high as 35.3 per 10,000 person-dives. The spinal cord DCS comprises 50% of clinical DCS and contributes 30% of long-term sequelae.

Clinical Features

A rapid ascent with full lungs and an obstructed airway from this very shallow depth could result in pulmonary barotrauma. Tissue rupture will allow gas from the alveolar space to enter the pleural space (pneumothorax), the pulmonary interstitial, the mediastinum (pneumomediastinum), and/or the pulmonary capillaries. The thoracic spinal cord is affected which leads to lower back or pelvic pain, followed by sensory loss, weakness, or incontinence.

Medical assessment involves evaluation of following factors:

1. Time of onset
    Onset of symptoms less than 10 min after surfacing could indicate AGE. Onset of symptoms more than 10 min after surfacing are more likely associated with DCS.

2. Profile of recent dive
   Greater depth and duration implies a larger inert gas burden.
3. Breathing gas
   Using nitrox within air exposure limits can substantially reduce decompression stress.
4. Thermal stress
   Excessive heating during the ascent and/or stop phase can reduce solubility in the peripheral tissues.
5. Exercise stress
   Exercise during the descent and/or bottom phase of a dive will increase inert gas uptake.
6. Altitude exposure.
   Flying after diving, however, increases decompression stress. A dive to 20 m (66 ft) at sea level produces an exposure pressure of 3.0 ATA. Returning to the surface at 1.0 ATA produces a threefold reduction in pressure.
7. State of hydration
   A relative state of dehydration can elevate the decompression stress.
8. Cold water dives—A cold ambient temperature slows nitrogen elimination and increases the risk of DCS.
9. Body fat—High body fat content precipitates emboli formation.

Vital Signs

Assessment of vital signs can prognosticate and dictate outcome of treatment.

1. Shock—It may originate from a cardiopulmonary DCS, tension pneumothorax, or hypovolemia due to physical trauma.
2. Cardiac and chest examination—Hamman's sign can be positive in pneumomediastinum. Diminished or absent breath sounds can be found on lung auscultation in pneumothorax.
3. Ear—Look for signs of middle ear barotrauma.
4. Neurologic and cranial nerves examination—To look for bends.
5. Skin examination—for bluish red rash over chest and back.
6. Joint examination—for pain only DCS.
7. Eye examination—for scotomas.

Altitude-Related Symptoms

The symptoms of mild mountain sickness occur after 6–24 h of ascent characterized by headache, nausea, loss of sleep, loss of appetite, fever, weakness, or dizziness. Severe AMS leads to rales, ataxia, and cyanosis, high altitude cerebral edema sets in followed by pulmonary edema at altitude exposure of >25,000 feet beyond 1 h. This leads to shortness of breath, dry cough with frothy sputum. The symptoms of spinal cord involvement are less common and symptoms of brain involvement are more frequent in altitude decompression sickness than hyperbaric decompression sickness.

The signs and symptoms occur with dives more than 33 feet or more. Joint and abdominal pain occur within 36 h. The most common sites of joint pain are the shoulder, elbow, wrist, hand, knee, and ankle. The characteristic pain of Type I decompression sickness usually begins gradually, is slight when first noticed and may be difficult to localize. It may be in a joint or musclepulmonary overpressure accidents can occur in depths as shallow as 6 feet. It presents as substernal chest pain with respiratory distress.

Arterial gas embolism mimics as a stroke. It can present as a pneumomediastinum. The nitrogen narcosis or rapture of the deep is reversible change in consciousness and neuromuscular function at depths more than 100 feet.

The bubbles lead to myriad symptoms of musculoskeletal pain called bends, bubbles in pulmonary or cerebral circuit. The mottling or marbling of the skin is seen.

Increased risk of nitrogen narcosis is seen in dives associated with alcohol, fever, anxiety, and hypothermia. Carbon dioxide concentration increases effect of nitrogen narcosis. The martini effect is positive.

Evaluation

A thorough neurological examination must be done to reveal brain/spinal cord involvement. A chest X-ray rules out pneumothorax. The clinical diagnosis of paradoxical air embolism is confirmed by early single-photon emission tomography (SPECT). Post gadolinium cerebral spinal fluid enhancement may be an early, sensitive predictor of blood–brain barrier disruption and impending cerebral infarct after air embolism. MRI performed in delayed cases reveal restricted diffusion affecting the cortical areas. MR imaging patterns of cerebral air embolism may show edema, infarcts, or gas pockets and facilitate implementation of timely treatment.

Decompression stress is commonly evaluated by scoring circulating bubble numbers post dive using Doppler or cardiac echography. Doppler only detects moving bubbles. Table 19.1 gives the scoring system for bubbles in venous gas embolism.

Table 19.1 A scoring system of bubbles in DCS (Echocardiographic)

Grade	Description
0	No bubble
1	<1 bubble
2	Several discrete bubbles
3	Multiple bubbles not obscuring image
4	Bubbles dominate image

The SANDHOG criteria uses a numerical score to assess the symptoms.

Dose of HBO

Surface oxygen should be used for all cases of AGE.

The principles of these US Navy treatment Tables 6 in DCS are:

- Recompression to depth of relief plus at least one atmosphere under 100% oxygen. In practice, this meant going to a minimal depth of 18 m or 60 feet for 5 min at 2.8 ATA.
- A maximum treatment depth of 30 m. This depth was considered a good compromise between optimal recompression of any bubble while minimizing nitrogen narcosis risk and subsequent decompression.
- Decompression phase at 9 m before surfacing and 2 oxygen cycles. Theoretically, this "overnight soak" was intended to allow all the tissues to saturate or desaturate to the 9-m level.
- The use of intermittent oxygen breathing during the last hours of treatment, i.e., 4 20-min oxygen cycles with short air intervals.

Total time duration is about 4 h and 45 min for resolution of bubbles and tissue repair. Table 5 is similar with short and less oxygen cycles (Total time: 135 min) for mild DCI.

Altitude-induced (hypobaric) decompression sickness (DCS) has long been treated with ground-level oxygen (FiO2 100%) and US Navy Treatment Tables 5 and 6. These treatment tables originate from surface excursion diving and, when implemented, require significant resource allocation. The aims of treatment are:

1. To reduce bubbles.
2. To prevent secondary bubble effects.
3. Promote oxygenation and reduce tissue edema.
4. Air breaks regulate nitrogen load.

If, after reviewing the patient's history, the hyperbaric specialist feels that the pain can be related to specific orthopedic trauma or injuryor altitude DCS, a Treatment Table 5 may be completed along with adequate hydration. Symptoms are relieved within 10 min at 60 feet.

Type II Decompression Sickness is treated with initial compression to 60 fsw. If symptoms are improved within the first oxygen breathing period, then treatment is continued on Treatment Table 6 (Fig. 19.1).

If a diver has had an uncontrolled ascent and has any symptoms, he should be compressed immediately in a recompression chamber to 60 fsw. If the diver surfaced from 50 fsw or shallower, compress to 60 fsw and begin Treatment Table 6. Table 6 can be lengthened up to 2 additional 25-min periods at 60 feet (20 min on oxygen and 5 min on air), or up to 2 additional 75-min periods at 30 feet (15 min on air and 60 min on oxygen), or both.

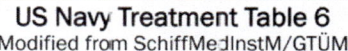

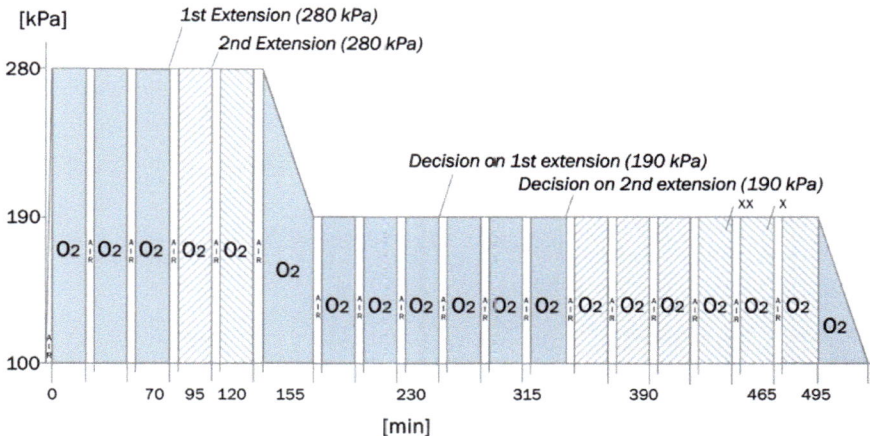

Fig. 19.1 US Navy treatment Table 6 for DCI

If the diver surfaced from a greater depth, compress to 60 fsw or the depth where the symptoms are significantly improved, not to exceed 165 fsw, and begin Treatment Table 6A.

The distance to the hyperbaric chamber can also be a barrier to expedient treatment. Emergency HBO$_2$ therapy with the Hart-Kindwall protocol in a monoplace chamber may be a suitable option for severe DCI, especially in remote locations with no access to facilities with a multiplace chamber.

Additional heliox tables at 4 ATA benefit a subset of spinal cord DCS due to a neuroprotective effect of helium.

The pressure is elevated to keep nitrogen in solution. Gradual decompression removes nitrogen from the lungs. Post treatment the patient experiences relief from dizziness and joint pain.

The patient is given repeated HBO treatments twice daily at 2.8 ATA (100% oxygen) for cerebral edema recovery. The recovery is good if given within 6 h.

Neurosurgery related embolism episodes respond to US Navy Treatment Table 6 (Fig. 19.1).

If HBOT is indicated in the case of inadequate decompression without symptoms, shorter treatment tables are possible, for example, "US Navy Treatment Table 5." Periodic neurologic checkups dictate treatment. Frequent lung auscultation and chest X-rays are useful to guide the protocol. Regular inspection of medical devices should be done during pressure adjustments. If severe neurological symptoms persist, a second HBOT treatment can also be considered according to the standard "US Navy Treatment Table 6."

Intervals between HBOT treatment is no more than 24 h, but no more than two sessions within 24 h. The treatment of children and adolescents should be carried out in an age-dependent manner. The duration of oxygen breathing depends on the severity of manifestation, the response to recompression, delay to treatment, the depth-time of the incident dive(s).

How to Prevent DCS
Avoid diving if obese, pregnant, have heart or lung problem.
Avoid excess alcohol or drugs.
Avoid flying after a dive.
Avoid repeated dives within 12 h.
Avoid cold before a dive or allergy.

Never hold your breath.

Discussion

Decompression sickness is based on sound clinical diagnosis.

Of the 447 cases, 83.2% had musculoskeletal involvement, 2.7% had chokes, 2.2% skin manifestations, 10.8% paresthesia, and 0.5% frank neurological features [1]. Hyperbaric oxygen treatment produced fully successful results in 97.7% of the cases of Type 2 altitude induced DCI. Only 2.3% of the cases resulted in residual deficit; no deaths occurred [2]. Gas embolism reported after ingestion of 33% hydrogen peroxide responds with HBOT [3].

Bubble detection by ultrasonic scanning of the heart can be used as a tool to assess the safety of decompression procedures for air dives [4].

Risk factors noted in 520 dives were repetitive dives, rapid onset, consecutive dives, and strenuous diving were noted [5].

Sixty-two mild and 39 moderate patients who recovered incompletely after initial recompression received additional 1–5 sessions of HBO following the first treatment. All recovered completely. In 124 severe patients who improved after the first recompression, 44 received 3 to more than 100 additional sessions of HBO therapy [6]. S2k guidelines for diving accidents emphasizes role of onsite 100% oxygen first aid, immobilization, fluid admimstration and telephonic consultation with hyperbaric specialist [7].

DCS severity scores have undergone a massive shift from Dutka and Francis score which included a timeline to Bossuges score based on assigning weights to neurological scores [8].

The BORG scale score for the diving group was 12.09 ± 1.04, while that of the injured subject was 13. In the DCS treatment, HBOT played a significant role in mitigating inflammation and oxidative stress, as observed by the reduction in 8-iso-$PGF2\alpha$, IL-6, IL-1β, and TNFα [9].

Three theories supporting 3 different pathophysiologic mechanisms of bubble toxicity: arterial occlusion, venous infarction, and in situ nitrogen toxicity. The nitrogen bubbles can interrupt arterial blood supply to the brain and spine either by direct obstruction of small capillaries or by activation of pathologic clotting [10].

Delayed hyperbaric treatment using US Navy Table 6 protocol trended toward a better clinical outcome with DCI. Late recompression for DCS, 48 h or more after surfacing, has clinical value and when applied can achieve complete recovery in 76% of the divers [11].

The definitive treatment of DCI is recompression and oxygen therapy in a hyperbaric chamber. The dictum is the sooner the recompression, the better the outcome. High flow oxygen clears the nitrogen pockets inside the tissues. Travelers who plan to scuba dive should ascertain whether recompression facilities are available in coastal areas. Divers should avoid holding their breath and breathe normally during ascent, which should be no faster than 0.15–0.3 m/s. The 120 rule in diving should be followed where depth of the dive (feet) and time spent underwater (in minutes) should not exceed a total of 120. This avoids risk of nitrogen narcosis and DCS. HBOT should be given as soon as a patient of DCS arrives as delay worsens neurological recovery. Multiple sessions are needed in Type 2 DCS with table 6 protocol.

References

1. Ryles MT, Pilmanis AA. The initial signs and symptoms of altitude decompression sickness. Aviat Space Environ Med. 1996;67(10):983–9.
2. Wirjosemito SA, Touhey JE, Workman WT. Type I altitude decompression sickness (DCS): U.S. Air Force experience with 133 cases. Aviat Space Environ Med. 1989;60(3):256–62.
3. Rider SP, Jackson SB, Rusyniak DE. Cerebral air gas embolism from concentrated hydrogen peroxide ingestion. Clin Toxicol (Phila). 2008;46:815–8.
4. Eftedal OS, Lydersen S, Brubakk AO. The relationship between venous gas bubbles and adverse effects of decompression after air dives. Undersea Hyperb Med. 2007;34(2):99–105.
5. Haas RM, Hannam JA, Sames C, Schmidt R, Tyson A, Francombe M, Richardson D, Mitchell SJ. Decompression illness in divers treated in Auckland, New Zealand, 1996-2012. Diving Hyperb Med. 2014;44(1):20–5.
6. Xu W, Liu W, Huang G, Zou Z, Cai Z, Xu W. Decompression illness: clinical aspects of 5278 consecutive cases treated in a single hyperbaric unit. PLoS One. 2012;7(11):e50079.
7. Jüttner B, Wölfel C, Camponovo C, Schöppenthau H, Meyne J, Wohlrab C, Werr H, Klein T, Schmeißer G, Theiß K, Wolf P, Müller O, Janisch T, Naser J, Blödt S, Muche-Borowski C. S2k guideline for diving accidents. Ger Med Sci. 2023;21:Doc01.
8. Boussuges A, Thirion X, Blanc P, Molenat F, Sainty JM. Neurologic decompression illness: a gravity score. Undersea Hyperb Med. 1996;23:151–5.
9. Mrakic-Sposta S, Brizzolari A, Vezzoli A, Graci C, Cimmino A, Giacon TA, Dellanoce C, Barassi A, Sesana G, Bosco G. Decompression illness after technical diving session in Mediterranean sea: oxidative stress, inflammation, and HBO therapy. Int J Mol Sci. 2024;25:11367.
10. KamtchumTatuene J, Pignel R, Pollak P, Lovblad KO, Kleinschmidt A, Vargas MI. Vargas neuroimaging of diving-related decompression illness: current knowledge and perspectives American. J Neuroradiol. 2014;35(11):2039–44.
11. Hadanny A, Fishlev G, Bechor Y, Bergan J, Friedman M, Maliar A, Efrati S. Delayed recompression for decompression sickness: retrospective analysis. PLoS One. 2015;10(4):e0124919.

Chapter 20
Hyperbaric in Ageing

Introduction

Ageing is characterized by lipid peroxidation, protein irregularity, and DNA breaks. *Drosophila* has been studied for longevity by varying levels of oxygen tension and proposed moderate hypoxia to extend lifespan. Old age contributes to death of organisms and mammals. Age-related diseases like diabetes and cancer are affected by growth hormone levels. Common pathologies in human ageing involve muscles (sarcopenia), atherosclerosis, neurodegeneration, osteoarthritis, eye disorders, and cardiac problems. Aging affects stem cells through changes in quiescence, differentiation ability, and interactions with their niche. Vascular ageing refers to changes in blood vessels with age. Extrinsic ageing is due to exposure to the sun which can be atrophic or hypertrophic. Intrinsic ageing is genetically programmed and affects everyone.

Etiology

Environmental (tobacco, pollutants, smoking) and genetic factors affect the lifespan of the human body. The lack of nutrients and stress plays an important role in reducing lifespan.

Telomere shortening leads to pathological changes in human ageing. The biomarkers of ageing are methylation of DNA. Ageing drives disease. Dermatoporosis is seen in both intrinsic and extrinsic ageing.

V. Mago, *Hyperbaric Medicine*, https://doi.org/10.1007/978-981-95-2644-4_20

Effects of Ageing in Organs

A. Muscles

   Sarcopenia is seen in old muscles.
B. Bones

   Ageing in bones leads to loss of mass, osteoporosis develops leading to Dowager's hump. The ligaments become lax and cartilage undergoes stress.
C. Joints

   Joints become inflamed and arthritic.
D. GI system

   Loss of teeth and gingival recession is seen. Liver impairment is common with decreased colonic motility.
E. Immune system

   Increases risk of cancer and infections with low grade inflammation.
F. Cardiorespiratory

   Increase in air trapping and dead space leads to dyspnea and chest wall stiffness ensues.
G. Endocrine

   A decline in pituitary and thyroid activity is seen. Abnormal glucose tolerance is increased.
H. Urinary

   Decreased bladder capacity, increased frequency of micturition.
 I. Skin

   Senescent cells increase and extracellular matrix in the dermis is damaged, leading to thin skin and loss of subcutaneous fat.
 J. Face

   Wrinkles, sagging, and loss of volume is seen over the face. The skeleton of the face suffers bone loss in midface and mandible.
K. Nails

   They become thick and hard.

Classification

Types of ageing
Biological
Psychological
Social

Types of Biologic Ageing

Metabolic agers
Immune agers

Hepatic agers
Nephrotic agers

Effects of HBOT in Ageing

Hormesis works in harmony to ameliorate ageing through oxygen. The alteration of oxygen levels improves the oxidant mechanism and prolongs ageing. Hyperoxic hypoxic paradox plays a central role in augmentation of mediators.

Upregulation and downregulation of genes plays an important role. HBOT inhibits telomere shortening which is a marker of senescent cells. Free radicals and scavengers are balanced to secure antioxidant effect. The levels of p16, p21, p53, lipofuscin, and SASP are reduced. Stem cell recruitment is potentiated, exerting anti-inflammatory effects and stimulating angiogenesis.

Angiogenesis plays a role in restoring capillary fragility and restores the vascular milieu of cells. This is facilitated by HIF 1 alpha due to hypoxia.

Age-related immune changes are reversed by HBOT by increasing HIF 1 alpha levels and ROS induced cellular damage. HBO acts as a hormetic entity which activates antioxidant and cytoprotective genes. Bone marrow stem cells are increased which hasten tissue repair. The telomerase activity is triggered with lengthening of telomeres and decreased senescent load. The cerebral blood flow is increased thereby enhancing memory, attention and age related cognitive decline. Improvement in skeletal muscle oxygenation enhances endurance and recovery. Improved insulin sensitivity is seen with HBOT. Collagen synthesis and wrinkle reduction is observed in the skin.

Discussion

HBOT plays an important role in physiology of ageing by increasing collagen density, elastic fibers, and number of blood vessels [1]. Another study demonstrated a decrease in senescent T cells whereas B cells increased after 30 sessions [2]. A single 90-min session can lead to respiratory burst, increase in caspase 3/7 activity and pro-apoptotic effect [3]. Effect of apoptosis is induced by caspase 9 induction and upregulation of bcl2 protein [4]. CD 34 cells increase 8 times on exposure to a pressure of 2 ATA after 20 sessions by stimulating NO synthesis [5].

Post-treatment values of HIF 1, 2, and 3 along with CD34 were raised after HBOT sessions with pressures 2.5 ATA rather than 2 ATA [6]. HBO increases memory quotient and regional homogeneity is improved in the left hippocampus, right inferior frontal, and lingual gyri, suggesting enhancement of cognitive performance [7]. HBOT can reduce fatigue in agonist muscles on repeated jumping exercises [8]. Low pressure HBO improves pain threshold, endurance, and functional capacity in physical exercise group [9].

HBOT improves memory, attention, and cognitive functions correlated with brain activity detected by SPECT in impaired cognitive function patients [10].

Patients with shorter telomeres are associated with early death [11]. A decrease in neutrophil ROS levels were observed after 2–3 sessions along with decrease in phagocytosis activity [12].

HBOT increases telomere length and decreases senescent cells in ageing. It improves cerebral blood flow thereby cognitive enhancement in aged individuals with decrease in neuroinflammation. Skin photoageing can be improved by hyperbaric therapy as ongoing trials are underway in paving solutions for looking young.

References

1. Hachmo Y, Hadanny A, Mendelovic S, et al. The effect of hyperbaric oxygen therapy on the pathophysiology of skin aging: a prospective clinical trial. Aging (Albany NY). 2021;13:24500–10.
2. Hachmo Y, Hadanny A, Abu Hamed R, Daniel-Kotovsky M, Catalogna M, Fishlev G, Lang E, Polak N, Doenyas K, Friedman M, Zemel Y, Bechor Y, Efrati S. Hyperbaric oxygen therapy increases telomere length and decreases immunosenescence in isolated blood cells: a prospective trial. Aging (Albany NY). 2020;12(22):22445–56.
3. Almzaiel AJ, Billington R, Smerdon G, Moody AJ. Effects of hyperbaric oxygen treatment on antimicrobial function and apoptosis of differentiated HL-60 (neutrophil-like) cells. Life Sci. 2013;93:125–31.
4. Weber SU, Koch A, Kankeleit J, Schewe JC, Siekmann U, Stüber F, Hoeft A, Schröder S. Hyperbaric oxygen induces apoptosis via a mitochondrial mechanism. Apoptosis. 2009;14(1):97–107.
5. Thom SR, Bhopale VM, Velazquez OC, Goldstein LJ, Thom LH, Buerk DG. Stem cell mobilization by hyperbaric oxygen. Am J Physiol Heart Circ Physiol. 2006;290:1378–86.
6. Heyboer M 3rd, Milovanova TN, Wojcik S, Grant W, Chin M, Hardy KR, Lambert DS, Logue C, Thom SR. CD34+/CD45-dim stem cell mobilization by hyperbaric oxygen - changes with oxygen dosage. Stem Cell Res. 2014;12(3):638–45.
7. Yu R, Wang B, Li S, et al. Cognitive enhancement of healthy young adults with hyperbaric oxygen: a preliminary resting-state fMRI study. Clin Neurophysiol. 2015;126:2058–67.
8. Shimoda M, Enomoto M, Horie M, Miyakawa S, Yagishita K. Effects of hyperbaric oxygen on muscle fatigue after maximal intermittent plantar flexion exercise. J Strength Cond Res. 2015;29(6):1648–56.
9. Izquierdo-Alventosa R, Inglés M, Cortés-Amador S, Gimeno-Mallench L, Sempere-Rubio N, Chirivella J, Serra-Añó P. Comparative study of the effectiveness of a low-pressure hyperbaric oxygen treatment and physical exercise in women with fibromyalgia: randomized clinical trial. Ther Adv Musculoskelet Dis. 2020;12:1759720X20930493.
10. Hadanny A, Golan H, Fishlev G, et al. Hyperbaric oxygen can induce neuroplasticity and improve cognitive functions of patients suffering from anoxic brain damage. Restor Neurol Neurosci. 2015;33(4):471–86.
11. Cawthon RM, Smith KR, O'Brien E, Sivatchenko A, Kerber RA. Association between telomere length in blood and mortality in people aged 60 years or older. Lancet. 2003;361(9355):393–5.
12. de Wolde SD, Hulskes RH, de Jonge SW, Hollmann MW, van Hulst RA, Weenink RP, Kox M. The effect of hyperbaric oxygen therapy on markers of oxidative stress and the immune response in healthy volunteers. Front Physiol. 2022;13:826163.

Chapter 21
Hyperbaric Therapy for Delayed Radiation Injuries

Introduction

Gaps in safety protocols and awareness has led to an increase in radiation injury in India. The radiation exposure in Mayapur Delhi in 2010 is an example of radiation exposure due to a fault in a Cobalt 60 machine. Exposure can also occur in industrial accidents and nuclear reactors. The coastal areas in Karunagapally, Kerala had background radiation from monazite sand. Pelvic radiation leads to bladder and bowel involvement with stromal, epithelial, and vascular damage.

Etiology

NRBC doctrine addresses the etiology of this condition, i.e., Nuclear/Radiologic/Biological/Chemical.

Acute exposure occurs after a load of 5000 centigray. The subacute injury affects the lungs after 2–3 months. Delayed injuries are seen after 6 months with exposures more than 6500 cGy. Healthcare personnel using radioisotopes are vulnerable. The various sites of nuclear reactors are another potential source of radiation. Alpha, beta, and gamma rays are responsible for causing radiation injury. Man made radioisotopes like Ir-132 emit gamma rays causing burns and death. The Chernobyl reactor explosion is labeled as a level 7 accident leading to thyroid cancers. Overexposure to X-rays in fluoroscopy units leads to cutaneous radiation injury. Industrial radiography is a source of X-rays and gamma particles. Risk factors are dependent on age (children and elderly at high risk), site of exposure (brain, spinal cord, lung and kidney more vulnerable), high radiation dose and treatment factors (poor technique).

© The Author(s), under exclusive license to Springer Nature Singapore Pte Ltd. 2025
V. Mago, *Hyperbaric Medicine*, https://doi.org/10.1007/978-981-95-2644-4_21

Flowchart 21.1 Outlines pathophysiology of radiation induced damage

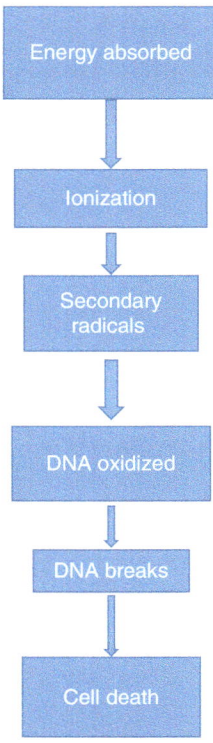

Pathophysiology

Tissues with a high mitotic index will be more severely affected at a lower dose, especially bone marrow, the gastrointestinal tract, and skin. The energy absorbed during radiotherapy manifests, as given in Flowchart 21.1. Direct effects of radiation are ionization of DNA and indirect effects are generation of reactive oxygen species. Key pathogenetic pathways involve vascular injury in form of endarteritis obliterans, fibrosis (activation of fibroblasts), stem cell depletion and parenchymal cell injury (neurons, glial cells, myocytes).

Epidemiology

Radiation injuries in the USA are mainly following medical procedures. Acute radiation syndrome occurs after exposure of more than 75 rad. Cutaneous radiation injury occurs at doses as low as 2 Gy. Annual cancer incidence in India is 79 per 100,000. The incidence of major radiation injury after procedures is 1 in 10,000. Prevalence of ORN worldwide is 5–15%. The incidence of Osteoradionecrosis (ORN) in India varies from 1–37%.

Classification

Based on INES scale:

Levels 1–3: incidents.
Levels 4–7: accidents.

Grades of cutaneous radiation injury:

Grades	Dose	Prodromal	Latent stage	Manifest	Third stage	Recovery	late
1	>2Gy	1–2 days	No injury	2–5 weeks	Not seen	C	Cancer
2	>15 gy	6–24 h	No injury	1–3 weeks	edema	H	Ulcer
3	>40Gy	4–24 h	none	10–16 weeks	ulcers		Ulcer
4	>550 Gy	Minutes to hours	none	1–4 days	nil	H	Cancer

Type and dose of irradiation is categorized as:

1. Orthovoltage—6000–7200 rads.
2. Supervoltage—6200–9100 rads.
3. Implant based—8000–14,000 rads.

Radiation sickness is dependent on two factors:

1. Absorbed dose.

   Absorbed.
   dose(Gy),
   Syndrome tissue involved.
   1–10 Bone marrow syndrome: leucopenia, thrombocytopenia
   10–50 GI syndrome: diarrhea, fever
   >50 CNS syndrome: cramps, tremor, ataxia

2. Rate of dose—criteria of dose is based on:

   <1Gy—low dose
   1–10Gy—moderate dose
   >10Gy—high dose
   Penetrating—X-rays, gamma rays, neutrons.
   Non-penetrating—alpha, beta.

Clinical Features

Symptomatology varies based on involvement of different organ systems in radiotherapy.

Acute radiation syndrome comprises several clinical syndromes:

1. Hematopoietic syndrome—occurs with a dose of 0.5–10Gy.
2. Gastrointestinal syndrome—occurs with doses more than 10 Gy.
3. Cerebrovascular syndrome—occurs with doses >50Gy and death within 3 days.
4. Cutaneous syndrome.
5. Neurologic— > 50Gy.

Clinical course is exemplified by the following stages:

- Prodromal stage.
- Latent.
- Manifest.
- Recovery or death.

Evaluation

A complete blood count is necessary every 6 hours to monitor the WBC count in exposed cases. The clinical outcome depends on lymphocyte depletion ratios. Testing for chromosomal aberrations in lymphocytes is done. Feces and urine collection is done to gauge radiosensitivity by Geiger counter. OPG is done to estimate the amount of sclerosis in underlying mandibular bone (Fig. 21.1). Colonoscopy and CT angiography helps in evaluating patients of proctitis with hematochezia.

The dosimeters worn during the exposure can provide an accurate measurement of the absorbed radiation dose. Laryngeal biopsy is diagnostic for laryngeal radionecrosis. Patients of radiation cystitis present with gross or microscopic hematuria detected on urine examination and upper tract imaging. The cystoscopy helps to reveal clots or bleeding points and take biopsy of suspicious lesions.

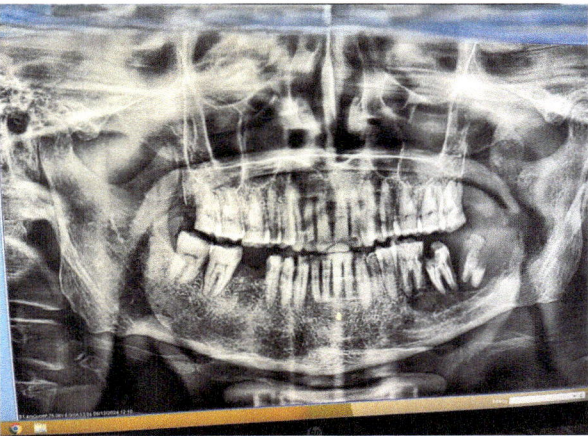

Fig. 21.1 OPG showing osteoradionecrosis with lytic lesions on left side mandible who received 20 HBOT cycles

The intestinal wall undergoes transmural pathological process after radiation, leading to stenosis and mucosal ulceration. This leads to mucosal hemorrhage intestinal fistulas, or perforation. Total colonoscopy is done. PET scan can differentiate between radiation necrosis and tumor.

Effects of HBO in Radiation Injury

ORN is common in mandible due to its density and poor vascular supply. It is due to hypocellularity, hypoxia, and hypovascularity.

Marx protocol is followed to treat ORN at a pressure of 2. 5 ATA for 90 min. Staging treatment protocol is advocated.

Stage 1—30 sessions for rapidly progressive ORN followed by debridement and 10 HBO postoperative.
Stage 2—radical debridement plus 10 HBO sessions.
Stage 3—mandibular resection is done.

HBOT helps to reduce complications in ORN.

Predisposing factors in osteoradionecrosis are enumerated in tabular form (Table 21.1).

Besides mandible, it can involve temporal region, ribs, sternum, clavicle, pelvis, and spine.

Soft tissue ORN involves cases of radiation cystitis, which leads to hematuria, nocturia, frequency or urgency. Ten sessions of HBOT have shown improvement in controlling hematuria in 11 patients in our hospital with resolution observed on cystoscopy (Fig. 21.2). Hyperoxygenation stimulates angiogenesis in the bladder by stimulating fibroblasts, enhances leukocyte killing and restores vascularity of irradiated bladder.

Symptoms of radiation proctitis like rectal bleeding improve by 41% based on various trials by its anti inflammatory effects and improving mucosal integrity. Good voice quality is achieved in Chandler stage 1 and 2 of laryngeal necrosis cases with hyperbaric therapy. The flap inset is improved after HBOT in radiation injury patients.

Table 21.1 Factors responsible for ORN

External	Infective
Dental extraction	Carious teeth
Surgical-Caldwell luc	Poor dental hygiene
Idiopathic	Candidiasis
Immunodeficiency	Periodontitis
Anti-angiogenic drugs	Diabetes
Xerostomia	
Smoking/Alcohol	

Fig. 21.2 Cystoscopic
evaluation showing
resolution of bleeding
points in hemorrhagic
cystitis case

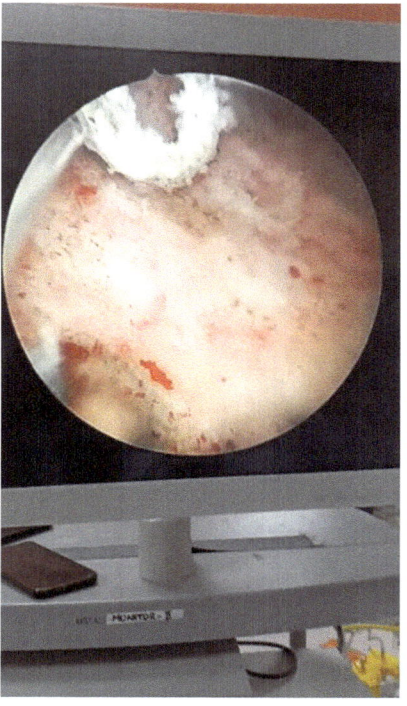

Cutaneous radiation burns improve with hyperbaric with partial pressures of 20 mmHg promoting production of collagen and fibroblasts.

HBOT exerts a neuroprotective effect in neurological injury post radiation. It exerts anti-apoptotic effects by activating bcl2. It stabilizes the blood-brain barrier and decreases myeloperoxidase activity along with ICAM levels.

Breast cancer related lymphedema of the arm and forearm is reduced after 10 sessions of 2.4 ATA for 90 min 5 days in a week. The fibrosis is reduced to a considerable extent. Improvement in pain is seen in all the patients. Regeneration of irradiated tissue is achieved with stem cell recruitment. ORN is treated by initiating osteogenesis. It reduces stiffness and pain after radiotherapy. It enhances skin graft or flap survival in irradiated tissue. Improvement in bleeding and pain is seen after 20–30 sessions HBOT for radiation proctitis.

Discussion

Late radiation injury causes lots of sequelae affecting the brain, gut, and blood.

Hyperbaric therapy plays an important role in eradicating Bacteroides melaninogenicus from gingival plaques in Chinese patients suffering from aggressive periodontitis [1]. HBOT is useful in reducing effects of irradiation on flexural strength and bone stiffness [2]. HBOT prevents the formation of ORN and prevents loss of implants in irradiated bone [3]. Complete healing of orofacial scars was noted in 6 patients and 4 showed complete disappearance of ORN [4]. Marx protocols promise 95% cure of ORN [5]. 12/19 patients received daily sessions of HBO 2.5 ATA for 60 min in severe ORN with good results [6].

Patients with radiation proctitis had improvement in healing of lesions and showed promising results in irradiated tooth cavities [7]. Pelvic radiation patients showed a reduction in LENT-SOMA score in cases of radiation cystitis and proctitis [8]. Breast cancer patients showed an improvement in pain, fibrosis, and shoulder movement after HBOT [9]. 84% of patients showed complete cure of hematuria in radiation hemorrhagic cystitis [10]. Seven out of 10 patients with radiation myelopathy and encephalopathy showed improvement in their symptoms after HBOT [11].

Cases of refractory radiation proctitis responded to HBOT treatment with 32% risk reduction and healing [12].

Late radiation injury patients are benefitted by its anti-inflammatory effect, improved angiogenesis, and cellular repair. It improves osteogenesis in ORN patients. Hemorrhagic cystitis patients respond with resolution of hematuria. Early initiation gives good results.

References

1. Chen TL, Xu B, Liu JC, Li SG, Li DY, Gong GC, Wu ZF, Lin SL, Zhou YJ. Effects of hyperbaric oxygen on aggressive periodontitis and subgingival anaerobes in Chinese patients. J Indian Soc Periodontol. 2012;16(4):492–7.
2. Júnior LHF, Limirio PHJO, Soares PBF, Dechichi P, de Souza Castro Filice L, Quagliatto PS, Rocha FS. The effect of hyperbaric oxygen therapy on bone macroscopy, composition and biomechanical properties after ionizing radiation injury. Radiat Oncol. 2020;15(1):95.
3. Hartmann A, Almeling M, Carl UM. Hyperbare Oxygenierung (HBO) zur Behandlung radiogener Nebenwirkungen [Hyperbaric oxygenation (HBO) in the treatment of radiogenic side effects]. Strahlenther Onkol. 1996;172(12):641–8.
4. Ashamalla HL, Thom SR, Goldwein JW. Hyperbaric oxygen therapy for the treatment of radiation-induced sequelae in children. The University of Pennsylvania experience. Cancer. 1996;77(11):2407–12.
5. Cronje FJ. A review of the Marx protocols: prevention and management of osteoradionecrosis by combining surgery and hyperbaric oxygen therapy. SADJ. 1998;53(10):469–71.
6. Maier A, Gaggl A, Klemen H, Santler G, Anegg U, Fell B, Kärcher H, Smolle-Jüttner FM, Friehs GB. Review of severe osteoradionecrosis treated by surgery alone or surgery with postoperative hyperbaric oxygenation. Br J Oral Maxillofac Surg. 2000;38(3):173–6.
7. Bennett MH, Feldmeier J, Hampson NB, Smee R, Milross C. Hyperbaric oxygen therapy for late radiation tissue injury. Cochrane Database Syst Rev. 2016;4(4):CD005005.
8. Andren J, Bennett MH. An observational trial to establish the effect of hyperbaric oxygen treatment on pelvic late radiation tissue injury due to radiotherapy. Diving Hyperb Med. 2020;50(3):250–5.

9. Spruijt NE, van den Berg R. The effect of hyperbaric oxygen treatment on late radiation tissue injury after breast cancer: a case-series of 67 patients. Diving Hyperb Med. 2020;50(3):206–13.
10. Cardinal J, Slade A, McFarland M, Keihani S, Hotaling JN, Myers JB. Scoping review and meta-analysis of hyperbaric oxygen therapy for radiation-induced hemorrhagic cystitis. Curr Urol Rep. 2018;19(6):38.
11. Valadão J, Pearl J, Verma S, Helms A, Whelan H. Hyperbaric oxygen treatment for post-radiation central nervous system injury: a retrospective case series. Undersea Hyperb Med. 2014;41(2):87–96.
12. Clarke RE, Tenorio LM, Hussey JR, Toklu AS, Cone DL, Hinojosa JG, Desai SP, Dominguez Parra L, Rodrigues SD, Long RJ, Walker MB. Hyperbaric oxygen treatment of chronic refractory radiation proctitis: a randomized and controlled double-blind crossover trial with long-term follow-up. Int J Radiat Oncol Biol Phys. 2008;72(1):134–43.

Chapter 22
Hyperbaric Therapy in Burns

Introduction

The incidence of burn injuries is increasing day by day due to primitive mode of cooking methods, fire cracker injuries, chemical and electrical burns. Electrical burns are very common in the state of Uttarakhand where workers or linemen get electrocuted by low lying high tension lines or electrical spark burns or due to faulty equipment. Chemical burns are common in factories or laboratories where high temperature molds accidentally spill over the upper limbs leading to deep burns. Various risk factors are involved in increasing the risk of burns, as exemplified in Table 22.1. Young children and elderly are more prone to burning accidents. Fire cooking accidents are common in females in rural areas and hilly areas where women still collect wood in the jungles and prepare food with open fire methods. The children are vulnerable to low tension line injuries due to low level of sockets and exposed live wires in domestic appliances. Dowry-related burn injuries are also common. Burns in males are involved in outdoor work, factories, house fires, and linemen working on high-tension lines.

Table 22.1 Risk factors for thermal burns	
	Ground level cooking methods
	Kerosene stoves
	Use of nylon clothes
	Fire crackers of spurious companies
	Combat injury burns
	Poverty and overcrowding
	Vitriolage
	Medical problems like epilepsy

Epidemiology

The mortality in burns ranges from 1,80,000 deaths per year in India. One million people are affected by burns in India. Incidence of burn deaths in children <5 years are more common in Africa. Hot water scald burns are common in the USA, where 3400 burn mortality are seen every year. An estimated 50,000 patients suffer from carbon monoxide poisoning in the USA.

Classification

It can be due to dry heat or moist heat (scalds).
Types of burns:

1. Thermal.
2. Electrical—high voltage vs. low voltage.
3. Chemical—corrosives or metals.
4. Radiation—X-rays, UV rays.

Based on Extent
Rule of nines—Body surface is divided into areas with multiples of 9%.

Lund Browder chart—useful in children.
Rule of palm—size of patient's palm is equal to 1% TBSA.

Anterior	Posterior	Total
Head and neck 4.5%	Head and neck 4.5%	9%
Upper limbs 9%	Upper limbs 9%	18%
Trunk 18%	Trunk 18%	36%
Lower limbs 18%	Lower limbs 18%	36%
Perineum		1%

Based on Depth
First degree—epidermal, blisters present.
Second degree—epidermal or dermal.
Third degree—full thickness.
Fourth degree—adipose tissue.
Fifth degree—muscle.
Sixth degree—bone involvement.

Evaluation

The evaluation of a burn patient is important to rule out other injuries or signs of inhalation injury. Severity of injury has been outlined by American Burn Association where major burns are 25% TBSA in adults <40 years of age, 20% TBSA in adults >40 years, and 20% TBSA in children <10 years. Burn depth assessment is done. Rule of nines is used to calculate TBSA burnt and amount of fluid for resuscitation is calculated by Parkland formula. Bronchoscopy is done in suspected cases of inhalation injury. Assessment of entrance and exit wounds is done in electric burn injuries and ECG is done to rule out arrhythmia. One has to check whether chemical burn is caused by acid or alkali. In suspected cases of smoke inhalation injury a chest X-ray or CT chest is done. The carboxyhemoglobin levels are measured.

Effects of HBO in Burns

HBOT in thermal burns exerts a lot of beneficial effects. There is a reduction of infections and immunity is boosted. Stem cell recruitment is initiated with a faster healing of wounds. It plays an important role in inhalation injury due to a reduction in edema and decrease in burn shock. Hyperoxygenation improves healing in penumbra of affected tissues, thereby reducing the incidence of complications. The fibroblast proliferation is increased with an increase in leukocyte production. HBOT exerts a bactericidal effect and potentiates the role of antibiotics like imipenems and fluoroquinolones. Carbon monoxide poisoning in inhalation injury is treated by HBOT where 100% FiO2 clears Carbon monoxide from the blood. A thesis performed in our hospital on 30 patients with acute burns ranging from 10% to 50% TBSA benefited with HBOT therapy in the form of improved epithelialization, decreased length of hospital stay, and improved angiogenesis on biopsy (day5). Procalcitonin and IL-6/IL-4 levels reduced with HBOT suggesting an anti-inflammatory effect. Figures 22.1 and 22.2 exemplify role of HBOT in promoting healing of infected ulcers over left side of face with a reduction in edema and healing of wounds. Figures 22.3 and 22.4 show importance of HBOT in healing after fire cracker hand burns over the dorsum of the hand. Infected right leg burn wounds with pseudomonas responded with good wound bed preparation and clearance of the infection after 20 sessions (Fig. 22.5).

Fig. 22.1 Left sided facial burns with loss of ear

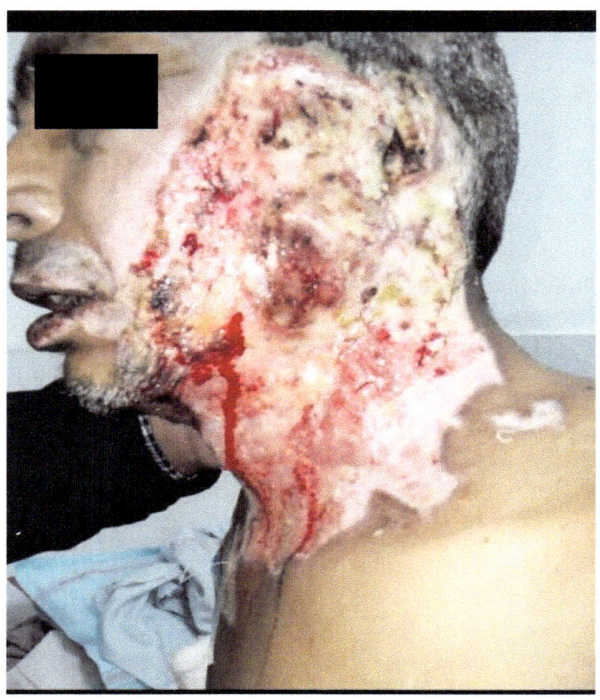

Fig. 22.2 Healing of facial burns after 10 sessions

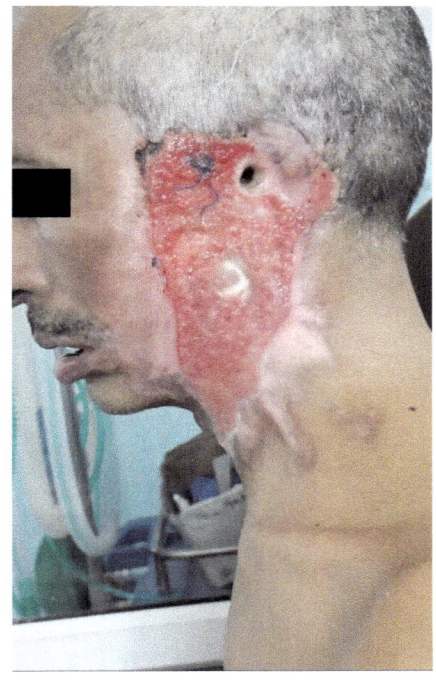

Fig. 22.3 Post firecracker
left hand burn over dorsum

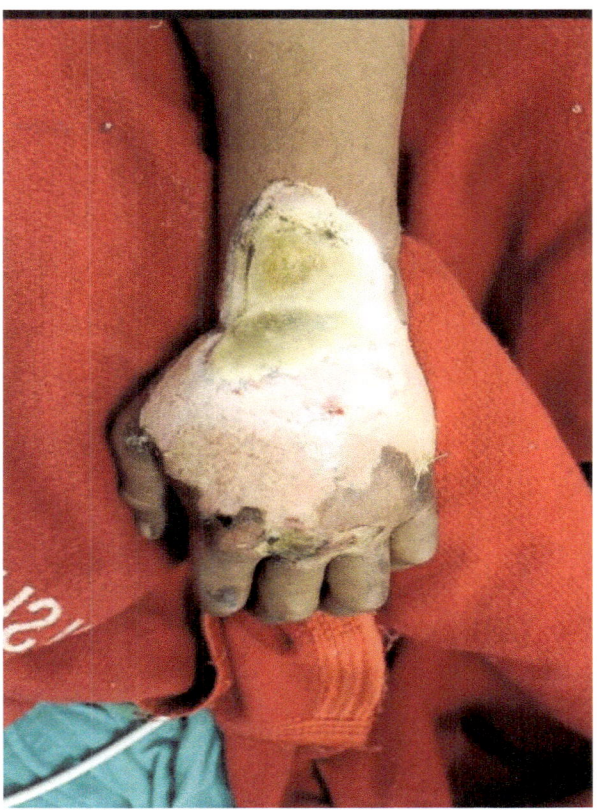

Fig. 22.4 Improvement in
healing after excision and
HBOT with healthy
wound bed

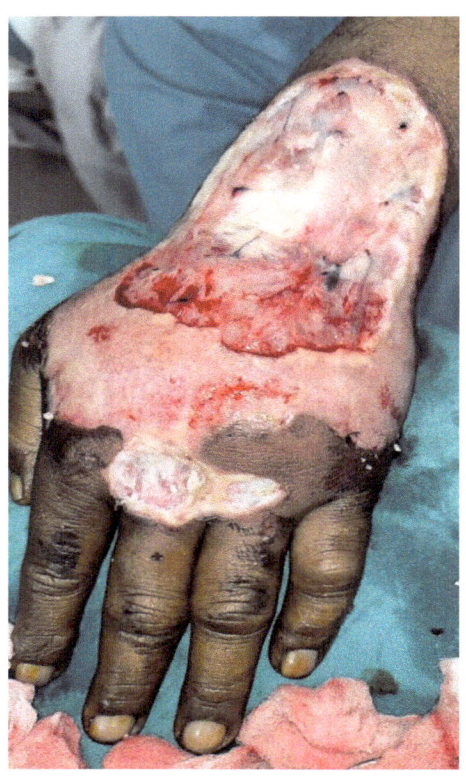

Fig. 22.5 Improvement in infected wound bed post burn right leg after 20 sessions

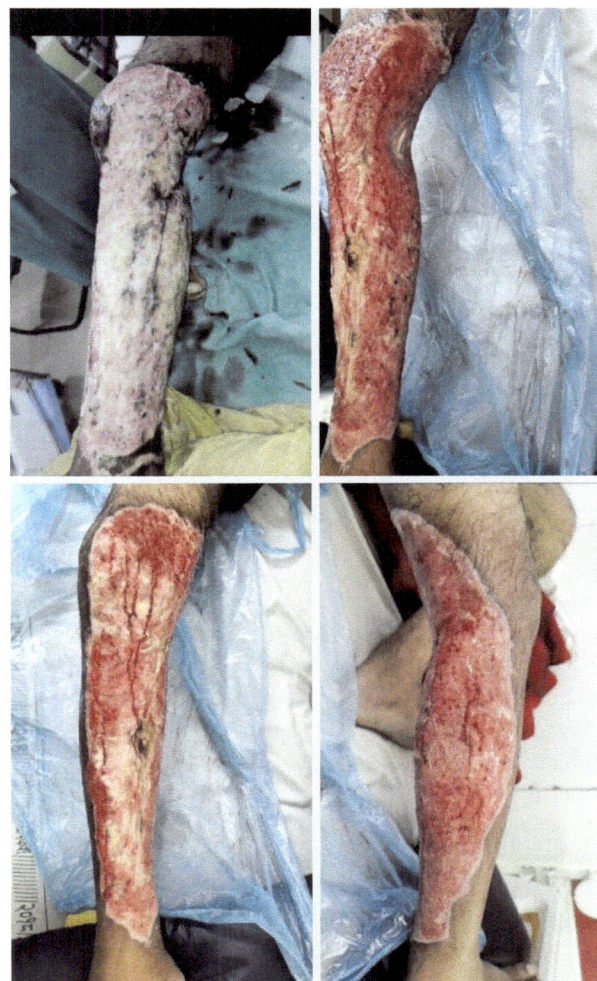

Dose of HBO

A pressure of 2–2.4 ATA twice daily for 90 min is the norm in the first 24 h after burns. The sessions can vary from 20 to 30 depending on the response to treatment based on healing of wounds. The surface area of burns starts healing and decreases in size after 5 sessions due to vasoconstriction and reduction in oedema. The thesis completed in our hospital has shown good to excellent results in 72 patients on histopathology with improvement in angiogenesis score and epithelialization of burn wounds. The length of stay was less as wounds healed faster with less complications. Ventilator support can be given in a multiplace chamber. The requirement of fluids is also less with HBOT. It improves leukocyte function by enhancing killing of bacteria. The burn wounds heal faster after HBOT sessions and limits secondary necrosis in marginal zones. It plays a role in inhalation injury by reducing oedema where an electric burn patient with vocal cord palsy improved after 5 sessions.

Discussion

Fire has played a dominant role in Hindu mythology where yagyas were performed since the time of Sushruta with herbs, oils, and fire. Injuries due to burns and their management by ayurvedic jatyadi oils are described in Sushruta samhita.

Dowry deaths due to thermal burns in married females is on the rise in India and is attributed to bride burning rather than accidental causes [1].

The authors reported a decrease in length of stay with burns and reduced mortality in their cases [2]. HBOT plays an important role in reducing infections, decrease healing times and fluid requirements [3]. There was a 42% reduction in wound hyperemia, 22% decrease in exudation and 35% decrease in size of the wounds with HBOT [4]. The authors stressed on the reduction of post burn pain along with improved healing with less infection [5]. Wiseman and Grossman propounded that effect of reduced tissue ischemia in burns lasts up to 4 h on completion of HBOT treatment [6]. Inhibition of HIF alpha signaling and mitigation of neuronal apoptosis are important features of giving HBOT in thermal burn [7]. Use of HBOT reduces the growth of bacterial organisms in burn injury [8]. The authors reported a reduction in levels of soluble interleukin 2 receptor (sIL-2R) and increased fibrinogen levels in 25 cases of >30% burns with hyperbaric therapy [9]. Patients with 20–33% burns were treated in a monoplace chamber at 2 ATA pressures with a significant reduction in length of hospital stay [10]. A large amount of air and heat reaches the lung in inhalation injury due to hyperventilation [11]. Eighteen patients had carboxyhemoglobin levels more than 10% and 5 patients reported ECG changes of myocardial injury [12]. Two hundred and thirty-nine pediatric patients with carbon monoxide poisoning (CO levels >20%) following burns were treated with HBOT and 189 showed complete recovery and 2 showed recovery with minor morbidity [13]. HBOT was given to 50 patients with burns ranging from 15% to 60% in a monoplace chamber with less pain score and fluid requirement and hospital stay was less as compared to control group [14].

After establishing initial goals of saving the life, protection of airway and hemodynamic stability, HBOT is useful in faster healing of burn wounds, reduce infections, reduce in fluid requirements, and decrease the length of hospital stay. This helps to attain an early vocational rehabilitation of burn patients.

References

1. Sharma BR, Harish D, Sharma V, Vij K. Kitchen accidents vis-a-vis dowry deaths. Burns. 2002;28(3):250–3.
2. Cianci P, Sato RM, Faulkner J. Hyperbaric oxygen for thermal burns. Undersea Hyperb Med. 2021;48(4):449–68.
3. Edwards M, Cooper JS. Hyperbaric treatment of thermal burns. 2023. In: StatPearls [Internet]. Treasure Island (FL): StatPearls; 2025.
4. Niezgoda JA, Cianci P, Folden BW, Ortega RL, Slade JB, Storrow AB. The effect of hyperbaric oxygen therapy on a burn wound model in human volunteers. Plast Reconstr Surg. 1997;99(6):1620–5.
5. Ikeda K, Ajiki H, Nagao H, Krino K, Sugh S, Iwa T, Wada T. Experimental and clinical use of hyperbaric oxygen in burns. In: Proceedings of the 4th International Congress on hyperbaric medicine Sapporo, Japan, 2–4 September 1969. Tokyo: Igaku Shoin 1970.
6. Wiseman DH, Grossman AR. Hyperbaric oxygen in the treatment of burns. Crit Care Clin. 1985;1(1):129–45.
7. Chen CA, Huang YC, Lo JJ, Wang SH, Huang SH, Wu SH. Hyperbaric oxygen therapy attenuates burn-induced denervated muscle atrophy. Int J Med Sci. 2021;18(16):3821–30.
8. Oley MH, Oley MC, Wewengkang LAJW, Kepel BJ, Langi FLFG, Setiadi T, Aling DMR, Gunawan DF, Tulong MT, Faruk M. Bactericidal effect of hyperbaric oxygen therapy in burn injuries. Ann Med Surg (Lond). 2022;74
9. Xu N, Li Z, Luo X. Effects of hyperbaric oxygen therapy on the changes in serum sIL-2R and Fn in severe burn patients. Zhonghua Zheng Xing Shao Shang Wai Ke Za Zhi. 1999;15(3):220–3.
10. Cianci P, Lueders HW, Lee H, Shapiro RL, Sexton J, Williams C, Sato R. Adjunctive hyperbaric oxygen therapy reduces length of hospitalization in thermal burns. J Burn Care Rehabil. 1989;10(5):432–5.
11. Watanabe K, Makino K. The role of carbon monoxide poisoning in the production of inhalation burns. Ann Plast Surg. 1985;14(3):284–95.
12. Williams J, Lewis RW 2nd, Kealey GP. Carbon monoxide poisoning and myocardial ischemia in patients with burns. J Burn Care Rehabil. 1992;13(2 Pt 1):210–3.
13. Aydin F. Hyperbaric oxygen treatment in children: experience in 329 patients. Diving Hyperb Med. 2023;53(3):203–9.
14. Kumar N, Tiwari VK. Evaluation of efficacy of hyperbaric oxygen therapy as an adjunctive therapy in the management of thermal burns. Indian Journal of. Burns. 2020;28(1):44–50.

Chapter 23
Ocular and Ear Complications

Introduction

The regulation of middle ear biomechanics is altered by dysbarism involving mastoid, eustachian tube, and tympanic cavity. This type of air squeeze is very common in persons who dive or board long distance air flights.

Physiology of pressure variation in the ear is altered as the volume of gases in a closed bony mastoid are distorted by their exchange between systemic circulation and middle ear. Eustachian tube blockade leads to middle ear barotrauma. This imposes distortion of tympanic membrane implicating pain, fullness, and hearing loss.

Role of hyperbaric oxygen in central retinal artery occlusion is promising but there are pressure and oxidative effects on the lens leading to cataract. Reversible myopia is also seen mostly after 150 sessions Early visual cell death and retinal detachment are seen as a consequence of oxygen toxicity. Keratoconus results due to an increase in ROS and oxidative stress. Glaucoma has been seen in a cohort of patients based on vascular theory amenable to HBOT. The nucleus of the lens is affected by oxygen toxicity leading to cataract formation.

Pathophysiology of Barotrauma

This depends on three factors:

A. Eustachian tube blockade.
B. Pressure dynamics.
C. Tissue damage.

V. Mago, *Hyperbaric Medicine*, https://doi.org/10.1007/978-981-95-2644-4_23

Eustachian tube blockade precipitates dislocation of stapes footplate with pressure on oval window. Further increase in pressure raises the cerebrospinal fluid pressure in aqueduct and leads to round window explosion. This phenomenon is seen in divers on descent. Similar is the cause of dental pain in carious teeth or fillings.

Inner ear decompression sickness results due to arterial gas emboli or de novo formation of inert gas bubbles inside vestibulocochlear duct.

On ascent, pulmonary barotrauma is seen due to over expansion of lung.

Etiology

Barotrauma is more common in patients with COPD, asthma, seizures, ear pathologies, and dental caries. On ascent, barotrauma is potentiated in air filled spaces like sinus or dental or ear. Scuba diving leads to barotrauma if a person ascends or descends too quickly. It leads to pulmonary injury.

Mechanical ventilated patients are at a higher risk of ARDS. Fatal injury to CNS can occur due to embolism once gas enters systemic circulation after barotrauma. Breath holding during ascent or decompression is a risk factor.

Types of squeeze in divers:

- Squeeze—due to descent in water.
- Reverse squeeze—ascent in water.
- Mask squeeze—failure to allow air into mask.
- Suit squeeze—due to air in suit of diver on descent.

Risk factors in barotrauma:

- Cysts or bulla of subpleural space.
- Scarring of the lung—trauma/infection/drugs.
- Airflow obstruction—asthma, COPD.

Epidemiology

The prevalence of pulmonary barotrauma is 50%. Incidence of barotrauma in ARDS patients is 6.5%. Middle ear barotrauma incidence varies between 8% and 68.7%. In India, Grade 2 otitic barotrauma incidence was found to be 47.4%. 500–1000 scuba dives occur every year in the USA and Canada.

Effects of Barotrauma in Children

Children are liable to suffer more from barotrauma due to adenoids enlargement, frequent Upper Respiratory Tract Infections and small anatomic spaces. Pain and conductive deafness is common during the compression phase.

Evaluation

Barotrauma of middle ear causes sudden onset deafness, nystagmus, and vertigo. Decompression illness of the ear is also seen but severe vertigo is seen in inner ear pathology. Maxillary sinus squeeze presents with pain over upper teeth. Air can enter subarachnoid space by barotrauma to the sinuses. X-ray of the chest detects pneumothorax. CT scan of the chest can detect bulla or emphysema or pneumomediastinum. Otoscopy should be done before every case scheduled for hyperbaric therapy with TEED scale. Eye examination is to be done by visual acuity examination, fundoscopy, and perimetry Raised eye pressures can be seen by tonometry. Abnormal values of data displayed in the ventilator, i.e., plateau pressures more than 30cmH$_2$O are found in ventilator-dependent patients. A proper dental examination is necessary before a dive.

Severity of Ear Barotrauma

Patients can be screened before HBOT with modified Teed classification to grade ear barotrauma.

Grade 0—No visible signs of injury but symptoms are seen.
Grade 1—Redness and retraction tympanic membrane.
Grade 2—Grad1 + mild bleeding.
Grade 3—Grade 1 + significant bleeding.
Grade 4—Hemotympanum.
Grade 5—perforation of tympanic membrane.

O'Neill is also used based on grades 0–2 with emphasis on bleeding, perforation, and erythema.

These grades help to identify patients suitable for scuba dives or flying. Ocular complications are mostly reversible myopia seen after 20 sessions followed by cataract seen after 150 sessions. Corneal odema and anterior segment ischemia is seen in sickle cell disease benefitting with hyperbaric oxygen.

Management

Rapid decompression at the rate of 0.1 ATA per second should be instituted if complications like loss of consciousness or seizures occur. One should encourage swallowing exercises or Valsalva inside the multiplace chamber. A technician inside multiplace chamber is always a helping hand to overcome anxiety and reduce barotrauma. During the session, if a patient develops tension pneumothorax an ICD drainage can be done and decompression is started. Patients of pulmonary barotrauma who develop embolization can be given US Navy Table 6 till symptoms subside. Monitoring of patients is necessary to avoid eye complications. Use of masks helps to curb eye problems like keratoconus and cataract. It lowers intraocular pressure in glaucoma patients. Hyperoxic myopia can be limited by giving 5 minutes of room air for every 20–25 minutes of HBOT.

Discussion

Barotrauma was observed in 18 of the 36 ears with HBOT after 7 days and otoscopy helped in identifying these cases [1]. Use of ear popper (pressure equalization device) helped to curb the effects of barotrauma and eustachian tube dysfunction [2]. Risk factors for barotrauma were observed in patients with abnormal mental status, hypomagnesemia, and hypoalbuminemia [3].

The authors found a high incidence in females older than 50 years, with 89 patients stopping their HBOT therapy due to barotrauma. 69% patients were Wallace Teed grade 1 [4].

Two hundred and sixty-two patients of otitic barotrauma were reported in patients with age more than 55 years, ENT problems, smoking, deafness, women, and altered tympanic membrane motility [5].

The authors reported patients who were denied HBOT if they were unable to swallow or do Valsalva's maneuver [6].

19% patients had otitic barotrauma after HBOT with Grade 2 barotrauma in 47% patients [7].

Symptoms were noticed in first 3 HBOT treatments and an overall incidence of 3.05 cases per 100 treatments done [8].

The authors stressed on a protocol that HBOT should be given based on rate of compression of 2 psi/minute [9].

Risk of oxidative damage to the eye increases during HBOT sessions using a hood due to increase exposure of ocular surface to oxygen [10].

Eighteen out of the 26 patients reported reversible myopia which varied from 0.5 to 5.5 diopters [11].

Large bilateral cataracts were observed in a patient after 46 sessions of HBOT therapy [12]. Seven patients developed nuclear cataract with decreased vision and reversible myopia was also seen [13].

Otologic complications can be prevented by teaching Valsalva maneuver to the patients or practice swallowing exercises before or during the sessions. Titrating the sessions with gaps can reduce incidence of cataracts and helps restore myopic changes in the eyes. The plateau pressures should be below 30cmH2O to avoid pulmonary barotrauma in ventilator patients. Use of masks should be encouraged in chambers to avoid ocular complications.

References

1. Karahatay S, Yilmaz YF, Birkent H, Ay H, Satar B. Middle ear barotrauma with hyperbaric oxygen therapy: incidence and the predictive value of the nine-step inflation/deflation test and otoscopy. Ear Nose Throat J. 2008;87(12):684–8.
2. O'Neill OJ, Smykowski E, Marker JA, Perez L, Gurash S, Sullivan J. Proof of concept study using a modified Politzer inflation device as a rescue modality for treating Eustachian tube dysfunction during hyperbaric oxygen treatment in a multiplace (Class A) chamber. Undersea Hyperb Med. 2019;46(1):55–61.
3. Lee JH, Lee HY, Sun KH, Heo T, Lee SM. Risk factors for middle ear barotrauma in patients with carbon monoxide poisoning undergoing monoplace hyperbaric oxygen therapy: a retrospective cohort study. J Clin Med. 2025;14(9):2984.
4. Nasole E, Zanon V, Marcolin P, Bosco G. Middle ear barotrauma during hyperbaric oxygen therapy; a review of occurrences in 5,962 patients. Undersea Hyperb Med. 2019;46(2):101–6.
5. Edinguele WFOP, Barberon B, Poussard J, Thomas E, Reynier JC, Coulange M. Middle-ear barotrauma after hyperbaric oxygen therapy: a five-year retrospective analysis on 2,610 patients. Undersea Hyperb Med. 2020;47(2):217–28.
6. Hwang L, Song M, Lee Y, Shin TM. Methods for preventing middle ear barotrauma in computer-controlled pressurization of monoplace hyperbaric chambers. Undersea Hyperb Med. 2019;46(2):107–16.
7. Saxena N, Raghavan D. A study to determine the incidence of otitic barotrauma during hyperbaric oxygen therapy. Indian J Otol. 2020;26(4):254–7.
8. Fitzpatrick DT, Franck BA, Mason KT, Shannon SG. Risk factors for symptomatic otic and sinus barotrauma in a multiplace hyperbaric chamber. Undersea Hyperb Med. 1999;26(4):243–7.
9. Heyboer M 3rd, Wojcik SM, Grant WD, Chambers P, Jennings S, Adcock P. Middle ear barotrauma in hyperbaric oxygen therapy. Undersea Hyperb Med. 2014;41(5):393–7.
10. McMonnies C. Reactive oxygen species, oxidative stress, glaucoma and hyperbaric oxygen therapy. J Optom. 2018;11(1):3–9.
11. Lyne AJ. Ocular effects of hyperbaric oxygen. Trans Ophthalmol Soc UK. 1978;98:66–8.
12. Hagan JC 3rd, Maturo JV, Kirby JP. Rapidly developing large bilateral cataracts in a 58-year-old woman after only 46 hyperbaric oxygen treatments. Mo Med. 2019;116(5):396–9.
13. Palmquist BM, Philipson B, Barr PO. Nuclear cataract and myopia during hyperbaric oxygen therapy. Br J Ophthalmol. 1984;68:113–7.

Chapter 24
Oxygen Toxicity

Introduction

Oxygen is present in the atmosphere in the range of 21%. Excess oxygen given at pressures more than 3 ATA cause facial pallor with cogwheel breathing. This is followed by twitching of perioral muscles. Beyond this level more oxygen leads to vertigo, nausea, and convulsions. These symptoms are aggravated by stress, fatigue, and cold environment. The pulmonary features appear at pressures more than 2 ATA followed by interstitial fibrosis, tracheobronchitis, and ARDS. This oxygen toxicity also leads to hemolysis of RBCs, aseptic necrosis of hip, and ocular effects like cataract and myopia.

Mechanism

The excessive formation of reactive oxygen species like hydroxyl radical, superoxide anion, and hydrogen peroxide disrupt electron transport chain through lipid peroxidation of membranes. Proteins are degraded leading to damage of mitochondria. Breaks in DNA are seen. The activation of NADPH oxidase in neutrophils leads to endothelium damage in lungs.

High risk groups for oxygen toxicity:

1. Infants and neonates.
2. Premature babies.
3. Bleomycin exposure.
4. HBOT.
5. Divers.
6. Patients on mechanical ventilation.

V. Mago, *Hyperbaric Medicine*, https://doi.org/10.1007/978-981-95-2644-4_24

Factors related to oxygen toxicity:

1. Pressure—normobaric or hyperbaric.
2. Time of exposure—FiO2 > 60% longer than 36 h; FiO2 > 80% longer than 24 h; FiO2 > 100% longer than 12 h.
3. Oxygen concentration—pO2 > 3 ATA(CNS); pO2 > 2ATA(Pulmonary).

Epidemiology

Incidence is 2% and seizure rate is 0.6%, i.e., 1 in 10,000 treatments. Barosinusitis is seen in 1 per 10000 treatments.

Presentation

CNS effects—Paul Bert effect is seen. First to appear are tunnel vision with twitching of perioral muscles. Tonic clonic convulsions.
Pulmonary—Lorrain Smith effect is seen. Reduction in vital capacity with absorption atelectasis is seen. There is a mild tickle on inhalation with coughing (tracheobronchitis). Diffuse alveolar damage leads to ARDS.
Ocular—Cataract, reversible myopia, retinal detachments, retrolental fibroplasia.
Bone—avascular necrosis of femur is seen.
Ear—serous otitis media, barotrauma. Barotrauma of ascent is due to compressed air which cannot escape in gas filled space. Barotrauma of descent is a result of decreased gas volume creating a vacuum in middle ear.
Blood—RBC hemolysis.

Management

Seizures—If a patient develops seizures during the session, one should remove his mask and pressures are to be lowered to 0.6 bar. Total duration of therapy should not be more than 5 h.

ARDS—One should lower the fraction of oxygen to 0.4–0.5 to avoid pulmonary barotrauma. Air breaks should be increased. Mechanical ventilated patients should be given FiO_2 less than 60%.

Pulmonary oxygen toxicity can be avoided by reducing partial pressure of oxygen. It can be helpful with frequent air breaks.

Deep divers should replace nitrogen with helium to avoid toxicity.

Ocular—Use of bibs in multiplace chambers are to be avoided if patient develops a reduction in visual acuity. Middle ear barotrauma is minimized by keeping rate of compression 2psi/minute.

Discussion

There is a reduction in vital capacity with patients subjected to HBOT in sitting position rather than supine position [1]. Hyperoxic acute lung injury is precipitated when FiO2 exceeds 0.6 and pO2 > 450 mmHg [2]. Pulmonary oxygen toxicity index is more sensitive to predict lung injury than UPTD [3]. Seizures in oxygen toxicity were seen in 6 patients out of 10,000 treatments [4]. The audit conducted in 8 out of 15 units in Australia revealed 33 seizures with an incidence of 1 in 222 at a pressure of 243 kPa [5]. An incidence of seizures was seen in 6 per 10,000 HBOT sessions and increase in pressure led to more seizures [6]. The ocular toxicity is not seen in divers as compared to exposures in HBOT patients [7]. The authors advocated eye examination for vision and perimetry before and after every session [8]. The seizures in hyperbaric therapy differ from hypoglycemic seizures in terms of revival in HBOT seizures on reducing oxygen but hypoglycemic seizures are fatal [9].

Prevention is better than cure holds true with this modality where reduced PaO_2 and frequent air breaks can prevent seizures during sessions. Ocular effects can be minimized by using face masks instead of hoods in a multiplace chamber.

References

1. Clark JM, Lambertsen CJ. Rate of development of pulmonary O2 toxicity in man during O2 breathing at 2.0 Ata. J Appl Physiol. 1971;30(5):739–52.
2. Kallet RH, Matthay MA. Hyperoxic acute lung injury. Respir Care. 2013;58(1):123–41.
3. Arieli R. The pulmonary oxygen toxicity index. Respir Physiol Neurobiol. 2023;315:104114.
4. Hampson N, Atik D. Central nervous system oxygen toxicity during routine hyperbaric oxygen therapy. Undersea Hyperb Med. 2003;30(2):147–53.
5. Sherlock S, Way M, Tabah A. Audit of practice in Australasian hyperbaric units on the incidence of central nervous system oxygen toxicity. Diving Hyperb Med. 2018;48(2):73–8.
6. Banham ND. Oxygen toxicity seizures: 20 years' experience from a single hyperbaric unit. Diving Hyperb Med. 2011;41(4):202–10.
7. Wingelaar TT, van Ooij PAM, van Hulst RA. Oxygen toxicity and special operations forces diving: hidden and dangerous. Front Psychol. 2017;8:1263.
8. Butler FK Jr, Hagan C, Murphy-Lavoie H. Hyperbaric oxygen therapy and the eye. Undersea Hyperb Med. 2008;35(5):333–87.
9. Manning EP. Central nervous system oxygen toxicity and hyperbaric oxygen seizures. Aerosp Med Hum Perform. 2016;87(5):477–86.

Chapter 25
Miscellaneous

Introduction

Certain indications have responded with excellent results where other modalities are ineffective. Chronic hypoxia is the leading cause in these conditions. The hyper-oxygenation achieved in a pressurized chamber overcomes these shortcomings and brings relief in signs and symptoms.

Vocal cord palsy

Paralysis of the vocal cords is due to nerve damage or conditions like electric burn injury, radiation and trauma. HBOT improves oxygen supply to damaged tissues and promotes nerve healing. One patient of electric burn injury with left sided vocal cord palsy improved with 5 sessions of HBOT at 2.4 ATA 5 days in a week for 90 minutes. HBOT reduces tissue oedema,stimulates neovascularization and improves nerve healing.

Fibromyalgia

Fibromyalgia is a disorder of multiple trigger points characterized by altered sleep, trigger points, fatigue, and cognitive effects. It can be due to genetic alterations, more common in women and aggravated with increasing age. This disorder is due to chronic hypoxia and abnormal brain activity. HBOT improves the delivery of oxygen to these trigger points reducing pain and improvement in levels of fatigue. Brain fog improves due to neuroplasticity and alteration in glial hyperactivity.

© The Author(s), under exclusive license to Springer Nature Singapore Pte Ltd. 2025
V. Mago, *Hyperbaric Medicine*, https://doi.org/10.1007/978-981-95-2644-4_25

Classification

Primary—no cause can be identified.
Concomitant—associated with some condition.

Epidemiology

The cases of fibromyalgia in the USA are about 2–3%. 0.5–2% population is affected in the Indian population.

Evaluation

Proper patient history, physical examination, and screening of associated conditions is necessary. The American College of Rheumatology score > 7 or higher of more than 3 months duration clinches the diagnosis. The symptoms are positive if Symptom Severity Score(SSS) >5 and Widespread Pain Index(WPI) >7. A sleep study should be done.

Dose of HBO

The patients are given 2–2.4 ATA pressure for 90 min in a multiplace chamber with face mask. Symptoms improve after 10 sessions as pain score improves and cognitive symptoms improve. Two patients from Norway and the USA were treated in multiplace chamber in our hospital at 2.4 ATA for 90 min 5 days in a week. They had an ACR score of 10 and responded well. After 5 sessions, both set of patients demonstrated a decrease in their pain scores and a decrease in their anxiety levels were also noted. Sustained effects are seen for 2–3 months after therapy. Sleep pattern is improved after therapy.

Lymphedema

Lymphedema in India is caused by the worms Wucheria Bancrofti which obstruct the lymphatics and induces swelling of lower limbs, breasts, and genitalia. Brugia species involves only lower limbs. This disease is spread by Culex and anopheles mosquitoes.

It can present as hydrocele, lower limb swelling, scrotal swelling, penile edema and elephantiasis. Breast cancer related affects the upper limbs leading to impairment of function and altered quality of life. The main risk factors in breast cancer related are number of axillary nodes removed and staging.

Classification

Primary—congenital hypoplasia/praecox/tarda(>35 years).
Secondary—due to known condition.
Clinical staging classification(Bruner).
Subclinical—no edema despite excess fluid in interstitium.

1. Edema pits on pressure.
2. Edema does not pit.
3. Edema associated with fibrosis.

Epidemiology

Higher number of cases are seen in India, Africa, and Indonesia. Incidence of breast cancer related lymphedema in the USA is 3–65%. 250 million cases are seen worldwide.

Grading of Lymphedema

Grade 1—Reversible pitting edema.
Grade 2—Pitting edema not reversing.
Grade 3—Non-pitting edema with thickening.
Grade 4—non-pitting edema, thickening and warty excrescences.

Evaluation

The microfilaria are examined by peripheral smear and ICT card test. Measurement of the limbs at fixed bony points to assess girth of the limbs and volume displacement by perometry is done. ICG lymphoscintigraphy is done to assess the stage of lower limb lymphedema. Bioelectrical bioimpedance can also be done to assess the volume of the limbs.

Dose of HBO

The patients with Stage 1 and 2 lymphedema are given 2–2.4 ATA 5 days in a week for 90 min. A decrease in girth of the limbs is noticed after a gap of 20 sessions and patient feels a soft compliance of the skin and soft tissues after treatment. The lower limb circumference was reduced by 2 cm in patients scheduled in our hospital with a reduction of pain after 10 sessions. Hyperoxygenation improves lymphangiogenesis with reduction of oedema and fibrosis in early cases. Most of the patients described a softer feel of their limbs after therapy. Risk of infection is reduced and healing of lymphoedematous ulcers is seen after 10–20 sessions. Post radiation lymphoedema show reduced limb volume and improved skin condition. Pain and heaviness is reduced after 10 sessions with improved mobility and function.

Long Covid Syndrome

Covid-19 pandemic has caused sequelae in the form of Long Covid syndrome with features of brain fog, muscle weakness, and fatigue lingering for 3 months. It affects young male persons with cough as predominant symptom followed by weakness. Patients who have received 2 doses of the vaccine are more prone.

Epidemiology

10–35% of the patients harbor long Covid for 3 months after SARS Covid-19 infection. Sixty-five million people are fraught with this syndrome. In India, 8.2% of patients reported with this illness.

Dose of HBO

Patients are given pressures of 2-2.4 ATA for 5 days in a week once daily by hood in a multiplace chamber. There is an improvement in Chalder fatigue scale after 10 sessions. This therapy improved the chronic hypoxia associated with this condition.

Discussion

The authors reported married females to be more affected with moderate depression and bodyaches in a cohort of 121 patients [1]. Four RCTs outlined excellent results with HBOT in relief of pain predominantly [2]. This study emphasizes role of

HBOT in reducing pain of trigger points by neuroplasticity and decrease in the brain activity of posterior areas on SPECT [3]. Ten patients of lymphedema showed an improvement in function, particularly compression therapy combined with HBOT [4].

There was >20% reduction in arm edema in 3 patients of radiation-induced lymphedema with HBOT, and 6 patients showed improvement in lymphoscintigraphy [5].

The authors found improvement in girth and 38% reduction in lymphedema of the hands after 20 HBO treatments of 2 ATA five times a week for 4 weeks [6].

The authors reported improvement of Chalder fatigue scale in women patients with long Covid of 3 months' duration [7]. This RCT throws light on the importance of improved brain cerebral blood flow in insula and supramarginal gyrus with improved cognitive, sleep, and pain [8].

HBOT holds hope in curing chronic conditions with increased delivery of oxygen at target sites, reducing edema and inflammation.

References

1. Ramteke S, Ramteke S, Yadav S, Chandak N. Clinical features, socio-cultural characteristics, sleep patterns, and depression in fibromyalgia patients from India: a cross-sectional study. Open Rheum J. 2023;17:1–8.
2. Cao C, Li Q, Zhang X, Varrassi G, Wang H. Effectiveness of hyperbaric oxygen for fibromyalgia: a meta-analysis of randomized controlled trials. Clin Pract. 2023;13(3):583–95.
3. Efrati S, Golan H, Bechor Y, Faran Y, Daphna-Tekoah S, Sekler G, Fishlev G, Ablin JN, Bergan J, Volkov O, Friedman M, Ben-Jacob E, Buskila D. Hyperbaric oxygen therapy can diminish fibromyalgia syndrome–prospective clinical trial. PLoS One. 2015;10(5):e0127012.
4. Koo JH, Song SH, Oh HS, Oh SH. Comparison of the short-term effects of hyperbaric oxygen therapy and complex decongestive therapy on breast cancer-related lymphedema: a pilot study. Medicine (Baltimore). 2020;99(11):e19564.
5. Gothard L, Stanton A, MacLaren J, et al. Non-randomised phase II trial of hyperbaric oxygen therapy in patients with chronic arm lymphoedema and tissue fibrosis after radiotherapy for early breast cancer. Radiother Oncol. 2004;70:217–24.
6. Teas J, Cunningham JE, Cone L, Jansen K, Raghavan SK, Nitcheva DK, Xie D, Butler WM. Can hyperbaric oxygen therapy reduce breast cancer treatment-related lymphedema? A pilot study. J Womens Health (Larchmt). 2004;13(9):1008–18.
7. Robbins T, Gonevski M, Clark C, Baitule S, Sharma K, Magar A, Patel K, Sankar S, Kyrou I, Ali A, Randeva HS. Hyperbaric oxygen therapy for the treatment of long COVID: early evaluation of a highly promising intervention. Clin Med (Lond). 2021;21(6):e629–32.
8. Zilberman-Itskovich S, Catalogna M, Sasson E, Elman-Shina K, Hadanny A, Lang E, Finci S, Polak N, Fishlev G, Korin C, Shorer R, Parag Y, Sova M, Efrati S. Hyperbaric oxygen therapy improves neurocognitive functions and symptoms of post-COVID condition: randomized controlled trial. Sci Rep. 2022;12(1):11252.

Chapter 26
Safety and Fire Hazards in Hyperbaric Therapy

Introduction

Since the historic times, these chambers have been made like Cunningham's domicilium which went into problems due to risks of uncontrolled or excessive pressure and these chambers were subsequently closed. There was a potential fire risk exemplified by the Milan disaster leading to 11 deaths.

The triangle of fire clearly gives an example why fire is a potential threat before, during, or after the sessions in a hyperbaric chamber. A closed pressurized chamber full of oxygen like the monoplace is like a time bomb which can explode any time if ignition sources are not non-combustible or there are undue generation of static sparks during the sessions. One cannot open the door of a pressurized chamber, so rapid removal of the patients is impossible. Smoke and other gases also pose a risk to the working of the chambers.

The SOPs of the hyperbaric chamber must clearly specify the objectives, working of the equipment, maintenance, incident reports, and safety protocols with quality controls for the doctors, patients, and healthcare personnel.

Fire safety drills are conducted every 6 months to educate the hyperbaric specialists, nursing officers, and technicians of the nuances of fire and methods of fire safety. The equipment has an in built deluge system which gets activated and sprays water if there is a fire.

Certain areas in the hyperbaric chamber are at a risk which should be marked to avoid mishaps and ensure compliance and safety of the attendants. Fire retardant material is used for making seats in the chamber.

V. Mago, *Hyperbaric Medicine*, https://doi.org/10.1007/978-981-95-2644-4_26

Safety of Chamber Equipment

Risk Factor Areas in Equipment and Consumables

1. Electrical fittings—These are periodically checked and exposed wiring are encased in fire proof materials to avoid ignition or sparks.
2. Clothes—The patients, attendants, and hyperbaric doctors must wear 100% cotton clothes to ensure safety inside the chamber.
3. Smoking—Smoking is to be banned in and around the chamber.
4. Shoes/slippers—Leather shoes are to be avoided inside the chamber. Patients and nursing officers must enter the chamber barefooted so that potential risks are eliminated.
5. Acrylic windows—The windows of the chamber are made up of acrylic to avoid risk of fires.
6. Implantable pacemakers or epidural pumps—Patients with implantable pacemakers can malfunction or get deformed. Epidural pumps do not deliver proper dosage of the drugs.

Risks in Critical ICU Areas

The infusions can be safely administered through suitable tubings in a monoplace chamber. The CO_2 readings are affected in a pressurized chamber. Certain life support activities like ECMO, dialysis, and cardiac assist cases cannot be performed in a hyperbaric chamber.

Duties assigned to a chamber operator or nursing staff includes control on the gases entering the chamber with proper pressurization and depressurization following safety protocols and keeps chamber climate at normal temperatures. They also maintain a duty log register of all adverse event incidents.

Dos and Don'ts Inside the Chamber

The oxygen concentration inside the chamber should be monitored with air breaks using air to avoid risks of oxygen toxicity. Patients can be encouraged to use bibs or hoods to decrease oxygen buildup. Bibs are built in breathing systems providing oxygen to the patient (Fig. 26.1) and an acrylic safety valve (Fig. 26.2) is used in the bib to ensure its fitting and leak of gases. This valve can get torn and needs to be replaced. The oral nasal mask can also be used to provide oxygen with a connecting circuit (Fig. 26.3). The mask can be cleaned or replaced after every session.

The chambers operated in our hospital are maintained and monitored by nursing officers who keep a check on patient's recovery and in-chamber protection both before and after the sessions. Every patient is acclimatized about Valsalva maneuver to avoid otitic barotrauma. Supervision is done by nursing staff to ensure proper

Fig. 26.1 Bib (Built in Breathing system) used in multiplace chamber

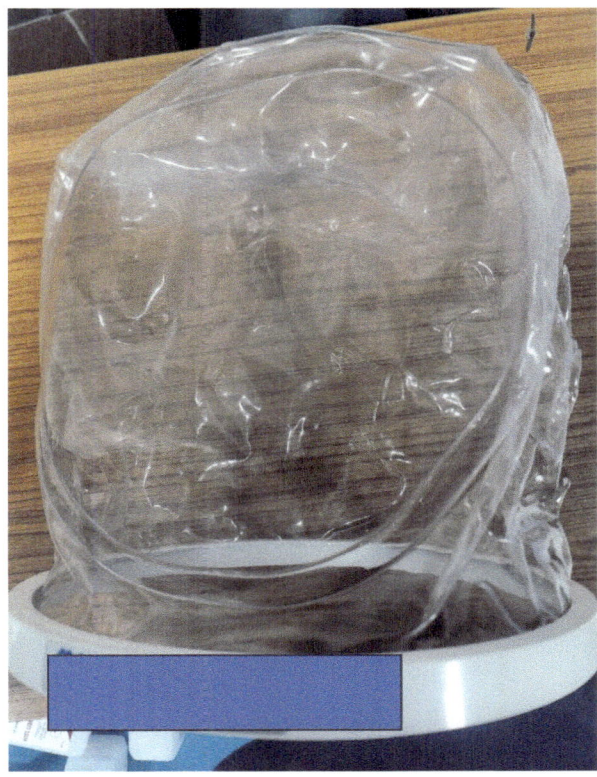

Fig. 26.2 Acrylic valve used in a bib

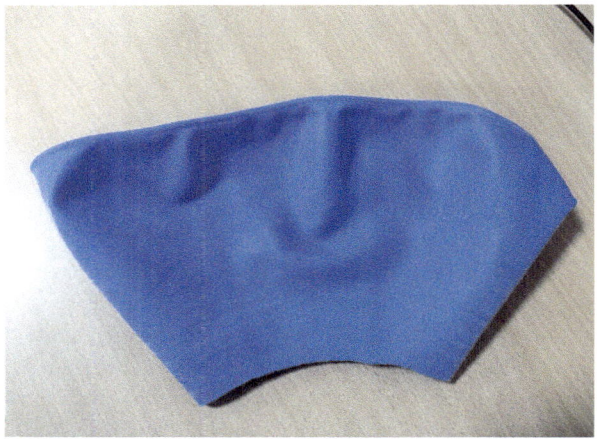

Fig. 26.3 Face mask with circuit

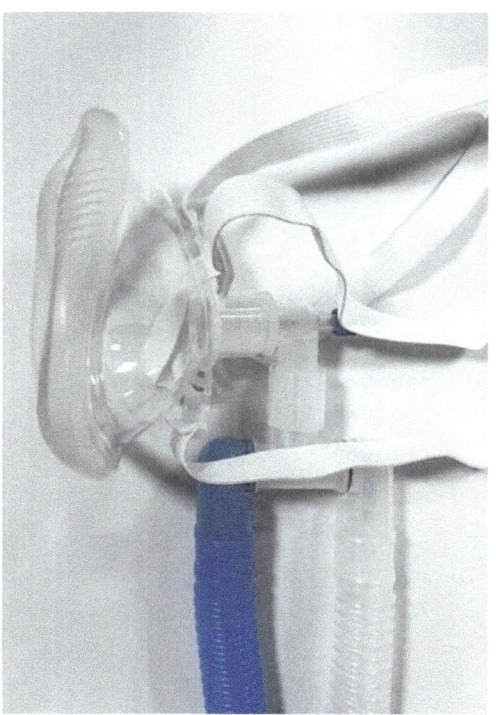

delivery of pressures and time of the sessions. Risk benefit profile is maintained in a proforma filled for each and every patient. The oxygen level inside the chamber should be 21–23% to prevent incidence of fires. Grounding of all the electrical chambers should be checked.

Intermittent breathing of air is instituted in cases of CNS toxicity. This decreases the incidence of seizures inside the chamber.

NFPA 99 document ensures guidelines for setup and maintenance of these chambers and needs to be followed. A safety protocol is also implemented through this document. This document ensures role of the safety director to minimize risk of fires. Hyperbaric chamber ventilation should be 3 actual cubic feet per minute (84.9 ALPM) to avoid oxygen pooling. The air quality requirements in any hyperbaric facility should be limited to CO_2 less than 5000 ppm, Relative humidity of 50–60%, CO of 5ppm, odourless and 0.5mg/m3 particles more than 5um.

One should avoid entry of newspaper or any sort of reading material. Medical gadgets are banned inside the chamber. Use of nail lacquers and hair styling gels are to be avoided. Caution should be exercised in patients who have implantable pacemakers or epidural pumps as they malfunction in pressurized chambers. Deluge systems are checked periodically ensuring storage of water in 2 tanks for any breakout of fire.

Pregnant patients and cardiac patients with ejection fraction of less than 30% should be excluded. There is an inherent risk of hypoglycemia inside the chamber so diabetic patients should be screened and routine glucometry should be done in all the patients. Parents should accompany children inside the chamber.

Sports diving injuries in coastal areas can be avoided by proper screening of the patients. The patients with asthma, COPD, or pneumothorax are contra indications for diving. Snorkeling and breath-hold diving should not be done in depths more than 30 feet or currents more than 0.5 knots.

Syringe infusion pumps pose a risk due to increased pressure, ignition issues, and tube compliance. Hospira plum A pumps are useful to deliver medications safely in the chamber. Low infusion has issues with delivery of drugs due to tubal issues. Ventilators compatible in high pressures are used especially Drager, oxylog, etc.

The multiplace chambers are better equipped to manage critical ICU patients as the equipment can be easily used inside the chamber with adequate room for extra staff. Monoplace chambers lack this facility. Defibrillation should not be done in a hyperbaric unit.

The disinfection of the chamber is done with commercially available neutral detergents like Sanizide or Whiteley which are used to clean the chamber surfaces and windows. Proper hand hygiene with mild soap is encouraged. Regular cleaning and disinfection are done after every session. Do not use alcohol-based hand rub in a hyperbaric chamber. Soaps with glycerin should be avoided. Do not use sprays, oils, and cosmetics in the chamber. The metal storage containers should be used. One should forbid use of paper or magazines in the chamber. Oxygen compatible lubricants are used. Gas burners, lighters, and matches are to be removed. Cleaners used should be odor free.

Discussion

Fire and safety of electrical appliances was added in the Code of Good Working Practice in 1996 to ensure fire safety [1] of hyperbaric chambers. The oxygen index of various medical tapes and wound products was studied to check the compatibility of these items in a hyperbaric chamber. None of these items ignited in the chamber [2]. Hypoglycemic episodes are more prevalent in type 1 diabetes mellitus undergoing HBOT and incidence was 1.5% [3]. Simulation techniques in diving and SCUBA can be incorporated in curriculum to teach clinical diving scenarios to potential candidates [4]. Scuba diving injuries like inner ear barotrauma or decompression sickness with gas embolism can be treated with hyperbaric oxygen therapy [5].

Four patients of barotrauma and one case of claustrophobia were noted out of the 106 patients subjected to HBOT in a tertiary center. The author emphasized the role of technician to obviate risks of therapy by teaching Valsalva maneuver and his presence inside the chamber reduces the anxiety [6]. The authors noted barotrauma was more common in female patients and children less than 16 years. They found middle ear barotrauma as the major complication in their series [7].

After an average of 52.8 sessions, lung function was found to be normal and patients with sensory loss around the ears had a high risk of perforation of the tympanic membrane [8]. Management of seizure in a monoplace chamber is difficult because of pressure inequality [9].

Hospira plum A infusion pumps can be used both in monoplace and multiplace chambers but low infusions should be avoided to curb compliance of the tubings [10]. The devices approved for use inside the hyperbaric chamber are 2 ventilators (Maquet servo-iHBO and Siaretron 1000), syringe pump (Pilot hyperbaric) and Haux/Corplus 3 monitoring systems [11]. Eighteen questionnaires were screened to reveal that 87% units used a cleaner for disinfection and advocated nonuse of alcohol-based cleansers [12].

Management of diving injuries are crucial in coastal areas as hyperbaric therapy is life-saving in these casualties. The technician in the hyperbaric unit helps in proper screening of the patients entering the chambers by confirming safety checks, indications, and pressures before the sessions. Fire hazards can be avoided by following the Dos and don'ts of the equipment. A clean workplace and hand hygiene practices in the hyperbaric unit helps to prevent infection. The nursing officers in our hospital have been trained to provide hyperbaric sessions in a safe environment with safety checklists in place. They provide in chamber assistance and assist in the operational process based on compression and decompression schedules.

References

1. Gough-Allen R, Abrahams J, Allen M, Elner D, McClue G, Middlebrook I. Guide to fire safety standards for hyperbaric treatment centres. British Hyperbaric Association Technical working party report. Aberdeen: British Hyperbaric Association, 1996.
2. Bernatchez SF, Tucker J, Chiffoleau G. Hyperbaric oxygen therapy and oxygen compatibility of skin and wound care products. Adv Wound Care (New Rochelle). 2017;6(11):371–81.
3. Stevens SL, Narr AJ, Claus PL, Millman MP, Steinkraus LW, Shields RC, Buchta WG, Haddon R, Wang Z, Murad MH. The incidence of hypoglycemia during HBO2 therapy: a retrospective review. Undersea Hyperb Med. 2015;42(3):191–6.
4. Paganini M, Mormando G, Savino S, Garetto G, Tiozzo G, Camporesi EM, Fabris F, Bosco G. Emergency medicine cases in underwater and hyperbaric environments: the use of in situ simulation as a learning technique. Front Physiol. 2021;12:666503.
5. Clenney TL, Lassen LF. Recreational scuba diving injuries. Am Fam Physician. 1996;53(5):1761–74.
6. Mago V. Safety of hyperbaric medicine in clinical scenarios. Ann Afr Med. 2024;23(1):1–4.
7. Hadanny A, Meir O, Bechor Y, Fishlev G, Bergan J, Efrati S. The safety of hyperbaric oxygen treatment–retrospective analysis in 2,334 patients. Undersea Hyperb Med. 2016;43(2):113–22.
8. Plafki C, Peters P, Almeling M, Welslau W, Busch R. Complications and side effects of hyperbaric oxygen therapy. Aviat Space Environ Med. 2000;71(2):119–24.
9. Huang KC, Hsu WH, Peng KT, Huang TJ, Hsu RW. Hyperbaric oxygen therapy in orthopedic conditions: an evaluation of safety. J Trauma. 2006;61(4):913–7.
10. Al Balushi A, Smart D. Safety and performance of intravenous pumps and syringe drivers in hyperbaric environments. Diving Hyperb Med. 2023;53(1):42–50.
11. Kot J. Medical devices and procedures in the hyperbaric chamber. Diving Hyperb Med. 2014;44(4):223–7.
12. Huart D, Henckes A, Cochard G, Zahar J-R, Baron R, Saliou P. Infection control in therapeutic hyperbaric chambers: practical inventory in France. Infect Control Hosp Epidemiol. 2015;36(11):1375–7.

Chapter 27
Telemedicine in Hyperbaric Oxygen Therapy: A New Horizon

Introduction

Telemedicine means practicing medicine at a distance. Web-based patient management technologies, including web-based messaging, video conferencing, web-based educational programs, have brought recognition. Telemedicine has benefitted hyperbaric medicine therapy patients who have limited access to doctors and paramedics. It enhances communication with the plastic surgeon. Telecommunication linkages are widely used in military services for connecting base hospitals to remote military outposts.

Wound care is a visual specialty which involves use of images for diagnosis and management. It involves travel expenses and increased duration of visits with prolonged waiting times.

Real-time or video consultation (VC) uses video-conferencing equipment to connect the patient, often with their General Practitioner (GP) or nurse with a distant consultant. Portable devices like cellular phones and Personal Digital Assistants (like laptops and handheld computers) provide inbuilt camera to capture wound's digital images, and computing and networking features to deliver wound care of patients at a distance. They provide immediate image access and direct interaction and it is possible to gain knowledge on its usefulness. Periodic evaluation of leg ulcers and wound images using cellular phones is practiced in patients receiving hyperbaric oxygen therapy.

Quality and speed of image transmission is no longer an obstacle. Chronic wound screening with cellular phones using mobile TM revealed a diagnostic agreement of 90%.

Numerous telemedicine systems, including store and forward, real-time and remote, or self-monitoring, are used worldwide for education, healthcare delivery and control, sickness screening, and disaster management.

Telemedicine use in wounds treated with hyperbaric therapy can help in decision-making aids, remote-sensing and collaborative arrangements for real-time management of recalcitrant wounds. Telemedicine is useful in elderly population with chronic diseases. These days healthcare apps like MD live, Amwell, and Mytelemed are proving essential devices in telemedicine. Remote monitoring of grafts, flaps and burns is possible with follow-up of various types of scars. Rehabilitation is provided for hand surgery cases and in craniofacial surgery.

Equipment and Accessories

The technological drivers required to run these services include:

1. Computing and information technology.
2. Network infrastructure.
3. Technology-led society.

Network infrastructure utilizes wireless and satellite technologies for Internet. This needs an aptitude and attitude to develop technology-based society. Nontechnological drivers can extend access to health care and individuals. This type of telemedicine is useful for seamen, astronauts and healthcare for travelers.

The three modes of access are video, audio, or text. Patient consent is necessary and the moment a person initiates a telemedicine consultation, it is implied. An explicit consent is taken by a health worker or caregiver.

The limitations of this utility is a poor patient carer relationship, technophobia, and poor relations in healthcare providers. Privacy, confidentiality, and informed consent are missing in relation to ethical aspects for patients. The administrative constraints are regular maintenance, upgradation of instruments and software. There is a need to create awareness among common people and healthcare providers.

The benefits of telemedicine in hyperbaric therapy include better access to healthcare as it reduces travel time and provides faster accessibility. The patients can opt for specialist advice when it is not available locally. Table 27.1 illustrates the utility of telemedicine in various sectors.

Table 27.1 Sectors involved in telemedicine network

Serial no	Tele education	Beneficiaries	Output
1.	Provider education	Teacher/student	Academic institutions
2.	Patient/family education	Patients	Online books, mobiles
3.	Tele dermatology	Pediatric patients	Live and store and forward consultation
4.	Teleresearch	Sample size population	Recruitment study patients, validation surveys
5.	Burn Unit Telemedicine	Burn patients	Treatment and follow-up
6.	Trauma telemedicine	Trauma patients	Management, triage, follow-ups

The results of tests and images are readily transmitted. The referrals and discharge letters can be delivered online. There is a better access to information, resource utilization, and reduced costs. ISRO telemedicine network in India is covering 100 hospitals all over the country with 78 remote and 22 super-specialty hospitals.

Types of Telemedicine

Depending on the discussion between client and expert, it is divided into:

1. Prerecorded/store and forward—Sending email is the most common method. It is cheap, easy to set up, and practice.
2. Real time—This is done by video conferencing. This can be used as an educational or research tool in advancing knowledge of hyperbaric therapy applications.

Both the above types are involved in the management of wound care settings with hyperbaric oxygen therapy.

It can also be divided by

1. RMP to RMP(Registered medical practitioner).
2. Patient to RMP—patient uses telemedicine to connect to RMP.
3. Caregiver to RMP.
4. Healthcare worker to RMP.

Barriers to Telemedicine

The barriers to telemedicine are:

1. Personal
   These include acceptance levels in patients and providers. The providers face technological problems, fear of using gadgets, and less centers for training. Awareness among elderly and of rural background makes implementation difficult. A correct diagnosis cannot be made while interacting digitally as it lacks physical examination. Image quality issues is a problem. Privacy and consent concerns is seen with video sharing.
2. Technological
   These are mainly related to high infrastructure costs. The cost of establishing a telemedicine program varies at an institute or PHC level.
3. Legal Barriers
   Physician–patient relationship has to be strong with proper definition of roles and responsibilities. The liability insurance is a must to overcome legal hassles. The storage of records is very crucial. Cross-border consultations can be a legal hassle. ISDN security, encryption, and hospital network are areas of concern.

Discussion

Digital image referral for skin malignancy and other cutaneous lesions is a safe and cost-effective referral pathway, significantly reducing the interval between referral diagnosis and onset of treatment for skin malignancy [1]. The Mederi-Nexus™ platform was used to simulate the real-life experience of the patient, the disease, and surrounding environment [2].

A pilot study using 65 patients in a plastic surgery department evaluated by photographic images in association with an accurate referral letter offered a significant reduction in OPD time and inconvenience for the patients [3].

Teledermoscopy holds a prominent role for melanoma screening as well as for the diagnosis and management of pigmented skin lesions. Easy and accessible mobile teledermatology and teledermoscopy are an easy applicable tool for everyone and may open the door for a new flexible triage system for dermatologists [4].

This study strongly supports the use of telemedicine to connect home-care nurses to a team of wound experts in order to improve the management of chronic wounds [5].

Patients with chronic diseases can be monitored by clinicians remotely without the need to stay in a hospital. Remote monitoring makes disease management easier for both patients and clinicians in terms of comfort and treatment costs [6].

The session timings and chamber decontamination procedures, utilization of telehealth services for initial patient evaluations during the Covid-19 pandemic, led to adaptation of the evolving model of healthcare delivery throughout a pandemic [7]. The importance of telemedicine in pediatric emergencies and disasters and providing access to pediatric care to remote and underserved populations is highlighted [8]. Advantages of telemedicine services to the medically underserved population is improved access for the rural and inner-city child, enhanced care through faster and more accurate online assessment with reduced cost to the healthcare system and the patient's family.

Telemedicine services help in making mental health accessible to all [9]. This helped in getting in-prison consultations for prisoners.

Pain medicine care can be delivered in a pandemic like Covid-19 by telemedicine [10]. It cannot be a replacement for physical examinations or therapies.

This study reveals relief of anxiety in patients who received hyperbaric oxygen therapy in Plymouth and Hobart as chamber assistant inside multiplace provides a peaceful and calm environment [11].

Elderly population of rural background exposed to technology which is familiar, usable, desirable are able to accept and adapt better [12]. SMS reminders for appointments in the elderly for HBOT sessions can be propagated.

National Telemedicine Taskforce, developed by the Health Ministry of India in 2005, has been developed successfully with various projects like the ICMR-AROGYASREE, NeHA, and VRCs [13].

Remote monitoring is an important tool in telehealth to enable specialists or superspecialists to impart treatment to patients in real time at both hospitals and home. This tool is useful for hyperbaric therapy patients monitoring, assessment of response to therapy and outcome assessment in a cheaper way.

Public health and emergency preparedness is another proponent for telemedicine research. Innovative simulation techniques like intubation can be taught online for remote areas with limited access.

Telemedicine offers benefits to patients with chronic wounds, osteoradionecrosis, burns, and avascular necrosis of the hip by regular follow-ups and treatment. It provides multidisciplinary care and enhances patient satisfaction. Speech therapy in cleft surgeries is done remotely. Follow up in aesthetic surgery benefits patients by keeping privacy and cosmetic consultations.

References

1. Tadros A, Murdoch R, Stevenson JH. Digital image referral for suspected skin malignancy – a pilot study of 300 patients. J Plast Reconstr Aesth Surg. 2009;62:1048–53.
2. Jones SM, Banwell PE, Shakespeare PG. Telemedicine in wound healing. Int Wound J. 2004;1:225–30.
3. Singh S, Stevenson JH, McGurty D. An evaluation of polaroid photographic imaging for cutaneous-lesion referrals to an outpatient clinic: a pilot study. Br J Plast Surg. 2001;54(2):140–3.
4. Massone C, Wurm EM, Hofmann-Wellenhof R, Scyer HP. Teledermatology: an update. Semin Cutan Med Surg. 2008;27(1):101–5.
5. Zarchi K, et al. Expert advice provided through telemedicine improves healing of chronic wounds: prospective cluster controlled study. J Invest Dermatol. 2015;135(3):895–900.
6. Jeong JY, Jeon JH, Bae KH, Choi YK, Park KG, Kim JG, Won KC, Cha BS, Ahn CW, Kim DW, Lee CH, Lee IK. Smart care based on telemonitoring and telemedicine for type 2 diabetes care: multi-center randomized controlled trial. Telemed J E Health. 2018;24(8):604–13.
7. El Hawa AAA, Charipova K, Bekeny JC, Johnson-Arbor KK. The evolving use of hyperbaric oxygen therapy during the COVID-19 pandemic. J Wound Care. 2021;30(Sup2):S8–S11.
8. Burke BL Jr, Hall RW. Section on telehealth care. Telemedicine: pediatric applications. Pediatrics. 2015;136(1):e293–308. https://doi.org/10.1542/peds.2015-1517.
9. Dinakaran D, Manjunatha N, Kumar CN, Math SB. Telemedicine practice guidelines of India, 2020: implications and challenges. Indian J Psychiatry. 2021;63(1):97–101.
10. Shanthanna H, Strand NH, Provenzano DA, et al. Caring for patients with pain during the COVID-19 pandemic: consensus recommendations from an international expert panel. Anaesthesia. 2020;75:935–44.
11. MacInnes L, Baines C, Bishop A, Ford K. Patient knowledge and experience of hyperbaric oxygen treatment. Diving Hyperb Med. 2021;51(1):72–7.
12. Bujnowska-Fedal MM, Grata Borkowska U. Use of telemedicine-based care for the aging and elderly: promises and pitfalls. Smart Homecare Technol Telehealth. 2015;8:91–105.
13. Chellaiyan VG, Nirupama AY, Taneja N. Telemedicine in India: where do we stand? J Family Med Prim Care. 2019;8(6):1872–6.

Chapter 28
Ethics and Quality

Introduction

Off-label use of HBOT has emerged as an ethical dilemma for practicing hyperbaric physicians all over the world. The ethical issues in hyperbaric therapy revolve around distorted informed consent, wrong use of healthcare resources, and conflict of interest. Informed consent is paramount in research trials like randomized controlled trials where patients do not know whether their choices will be chosen by a random process and not promised confirmed proposed therapy. Key issues in placebo therapy are issues related to definitive medications indicated for particular disorder like schizophrenia. It contemplates the principle of equipoise.

Categories of Principles of Ethical Trials

1. Ethical inquiry of scientific content—Duty to society is obligatory.
2. Ethical conduct—Integrity and nondiscrimination.
3. Ethical treatment—proper informed consent.

Ethical and Quality Issues in HBOT

It can be:

1. Access to patients—Easy Access to the machine often is hindered by miscommunication.
2. Health issues—Patients with comorbidities are shunted for sessions without proper PAC checkups.

V. Mago, *Hyperbaric Medicine*, https://doi.org/10.1007/978-981-95-2644-4_28

3. Boundaries of therapy—Uppsala code has to be followed where a work has to be stopped if it is unethical.

The welfare of the research subjects in any trial related to HBOT should be based on the principle of beneficence. If effective treatment is present, placebos should be avoided.

The Declaration of Helsinki should not be violated. It is the responsibility of the principal investigator to prevent any harm occurring to the patient during HBOT sessions. Big data should be used with suspicion especially available on public domains.

Conflicts of interest are created in pharmaceutical sponsored trials where nobody knows the context of how, what, and when will the results be published. The best defined ethical principle till date is informed consent, especially of vulnerable groups like prisoners, children, and neonates. Ethical deficiencies are present between informed consent and duty to society. This holds true in the use of experimental drugs for cancer patients or terminal patients. Fabrication of data, falsification of results, and omission should be avoided in clinical trials with HBOT. Human rights should not be violated without racial discrimination. Availability of medical devices mandates its affordability and realistic values. Privacy and confidential use of public data is important in research. Knowledge, training, and awareness of researchers is paramount in principles of HBOT. Patients must be fully informed about its indications via an informed consent outlining risks and alternatives. The vulnerable groups like children and elderly should be counselled properly based on evidence based medicine and clinical guidelines. Socioeconomic bias should be avoided and patient selection should be based on sound guidelines and not experimentation. Quality issues should include chamber maintenance in the form of door leaks, leaks in equipment chambers and pressure gauge malfunction. The contamination and flow rate of oxygen delivery system should be checked periodically. A periodic surveillance of fire safety equipment and deluge systems is mandatory. Annual maintenance of equipment is needed to ensure a quality check and log maintenance for any incident report or adverse event. Protocol ambiguity can be checked by ensuring proper pressure levels based on the indications and keep a check on duration and frequency of sessions with air breaks to decrease side effects.

Quality of Life in HBOT

Improvement in quality of life has been observed in patients of avascular necrosis of hip, chronic osteomyelitis, and mucormycosis in our hospital. There has been a dramatic decrease in pain in patients with avascular necrosis of the hip and mucormycosis. The patients of osteoradionecrosis also show improvement in their quality of life after 20 sessions. The patients of fibromyalgia in our series reported an improvement in pain over their trigger points with a decrease in levels of anxiety and suicidal tendencies. A sense of well-being is noted in these patients. Venous ulcer patients often visit more than one center but are not satisfied but HBOT leads to an improvement in pain scores and speeds up healing of these ulcers. Poor patient preparation without proper protocols entails a high risk on safety of the patient. Telemedicine sessions performed in our hospital have shown a positive feedback of this therapy in terms of quality of life, decreased costs, and high satisfaction rates. Regular refresher training schedules and fire safety drills are important for treating doctors,nursing officers and health personnel. Patient related quality issues can be addressed by proper consent, pre treatment preparation and ensuring proper time-line of sessions.

Discussion

The problem faced by the hyperbaric fraternity is the skewed nature of evidence available and scattering of data [1]. The authors found a lot of pitfalls in this poorly designed study based on the assessment of primary outcome done by a vascular surgeon in diabetic foot plus remote data was used to assess patients by photographs [2]. Ethical issues are more common in unestablished indications incurring false hopes and expenditure involved [3]. New HBOT protocols can be made by design-ing better RCTs to define its role in breast aesthetics and abdominoplasty [4]. The placebo effect has now emerged as a form of sham treatment in HBOT where 131 kPa is considered treatment option rather than placebo [5]. Previous studies kept TBI and PTSD as off-label indications, but today these 2 conditions respond well with HBOT [6]. The obstacles faced in developing guidelines are lack of evi-dence, lack of harmony among experts, and infrequent computer-based reminders [7]. Large equivalence trials with waxing waning course and spontaneous remis-sions are the criteria for a placebo-based trial [8]. Proper SOPs outlining valid indi-cations to the patients and informed consent are the pillars for ethical trials in HBOT [9]. Recorded data should be destroyed in interviews creating ethical issues as data can be morphed [10]. The five things every clinician involved in ICU care using artificial intelligence ethics are to mitigate bias, appraise evidence, build trust, assess training data, and know how it works [11]. Nobody discussed the exposure of DCI in controls in an RCT performed for DCI treatment with HBOT [12]. The authors propound a 30-day delay after treatment in patient selection to achieve results in class 2 medical devices [13].

The unethical issues related to HBOT research which should be avoided are wrong selection of sampling method, wrong research protocol, and wrong control group. Low sample sizes cannot detect a true effect. 'First do no harm' should be the norm. Strict protocol adherence, pre treatment screening and emergency prepared-ness are the norms for ensuring quality of hyperbaric chamber.

References

1. Bennett MH. Randomized controlled trials in diving and hyperbaric medicine. Undersea Hyperb Med. 2013;40(5):419–38.
2. Mutluoglu M, Uzun G, Bennett M, Germonpré P, Smart D, Mathieu D. Poorly designed research does not help clarify the role of hyperbaric oxygen in the treatment of chronic diabetic foot ulcers. Diving Hyperb Med. 2016;46(3):133–4.
3. Mitchell SJ, Bennett MH. Unestablished indications for hyperbaric oxygen therapy. Diving Hyperb Med. 2014;44(4):228–34.
4. Mortada H, González JE, Husseiny YM, Al Jabbar I, Sultan F, Alrobaiea S, Neel OF. Efficacy of hyperbaric oxygen therapy as an adjunct in aesthetic surgery: a systematic review and meta-analysis of postoperative outcomes and complications. Aesth Plast Surg. 2025;49(9):2498–512.
5. Bennett MH. Hyperbaric medicine and the placebo effect. Diving Hyperb Med. 2014;44(4):235–40.
6. Hooker JS. Hyperbaric oxygen therapy: using evidence-based medicine to heal injured brain tissue. N C Med J. 2016;77(1):69–70.
7. Zielstorff RD. Online practice guidelines: issues, obstacles, and future prospects. J Am Med Inform Assoc. 1998;5(3):227–36.
8. Emanuel EJ, Miller FG. The ethics of placebo-controlled trials–a middle ground. N Engl J Med. 2001;345(12):915–9.
9. Chan EC, Brody B. Ethical dilemmas in hyperbaric medicine. Undersea Hyperb Med. 2001;28(3):123–30.
10. Dicicco-Bloom B, Crabtree BF. The qualitative research interview. Med Educ. 2006;40(4):314–21.
11. Shaw JA, Sethi N, Block BL. Five things every clinician should know about AI ethics in intensive care. Intensive Care Med. 2021;47(2):157–9.
12. Fife CE, Eckert KA, Workman WT. Ethical issues, standards and quality control in practice of hyperbaric medicine. In: Jain KK, editor. Textbook of hyperbaric medicine. 6th ed. New York: Springer; 2016.
13. Fife CE, Eckert KA, Carter MJ. An update on the appropriate role for hyperbaric oxygen: indications and evidence. Plast Reconstr Surg. 2016;138(3 Suppl):107S–16S.